NATURAL HAIR CARE *and* BRAIDING

Online Services

Milady Online

To access a wide variety of Milady products and services on the World Wide Web,
point your browser to:

       http://www.milady.com

Delmar Online

To access a wide variety of Delmar products and services on the World Wide Web,
point your browser to:

       http://www.delmar.com
       or email: info@delmar.com

thomson.com

To access International Thomson Publishing's
home site for information on more than 34 publishers
and 20,000 products, point your browser to:

       http://www.thomson.com
       or email: findit@kiosk.thomson.com

A service of **I T P**®

NATURAL HAIR CARE and BRAIDING

BY

DIANE CAROL BAILEY

ASSISTANT EDITOR: SONENI B. SMITH

MILADY

™

THOMSON LEARNING

Africa • Australia • Canada • Denmark • Japan • Mexico • New Zealand • Philippines
Puerto Rico • Singapore • Spain • United Kingdom • United States

NOTICE TO THE READER

Cover and Insert Design: Spiral Design Studio

Milady Staff:
Publisher: Gordon Miller
Acquisitions Editor: Joseph Miranda
Project Editor: NancyJean Downey
Production Manager: Brian Yacur
Art/Design Production Coordinator: Suzanne Nelson

Printed in Canada
5 6 7 8 9 10 11 XXX 03 02

For more information, contact Milady, 3 Columbia Circle, PO Box 15015, Albany, NY 12212-0515; or find us on the World Wide Web at http://www.Milady.com

Library of Congress Cataloging-in-Publication Data

Bailey, Diane C.
    Natural hair care and braiding / Diane C. Bailey; assistant editor Soneni B. Smith.
      p.   cm.
    Includes bibliographical references and index.
    ISBN: 1-56253-316-9
    1. Hairdressing. 2. Hair—Care and hygiene. 3. Braids (Hairdressing) I. Smith, Soneni B. II. Title.
TT957.B29   1997   97-25161
646.7'24—dc21   CIP

CONTENTS

CHAPTER 4

The Professional Consultation 47

CHAPTER 5

How Hair Types and Structures Differ 59

CHAPTER 6

Hair and Scalp Diseases and Disorders 73

CHAPTER 7

Basic Anatomy, Physiology, and Nutrition 97

CHAPTER 8

Shampoos, Conditioners, Herbal Treatments and Rinses 111

CHAPTER 9 — Textured Hair is Manageable 167

CHAPTER 10 — Braiding and Sculpting Techniques 181

CREDITS

Photographer: Preston Phillips
Accessories: Celestine Lee of Celestine Collection
                      Marion Williams—Deva by Marion Williams

Cover

Stylists: Diane Bailey and Fanta Kaba of Tendrils, Brooklyn, New York
Makeup Artist: Roxanna Floyd
Models: Awa Sane and Nina Nesbitt
Dresses (Fashion Stylist): Montgomery Harris

Cover Inset

Stylist: Diane Bailey
Makeup: Anthony Jones
Model: Judy Alanna
Designer/Stylist: Montgomery Harris

Color Photo Credits and Captions

1. African Kurl—Twist Out
   Stylist: Diane Bailey
   Makeup: Anthony Jones
   Model: Judy Alanna
   Designer/Stylist: Montgomery Harris

2. Silky Twist (left) and Texturizing Locks (right)
   Stylist: Lock: Diane Bailey of Tendrils
   Twist: N'gone Sow of Soween Braids
   Makeup: Juanita Diaz
   Models: Tammie Anderson, Sally Toussaint

3a. Crimped Single Braids
3b. Crimped Singles—Profile
3c. Crimped Singles—Updo
   Stylist: Susan Bishop of Jaka Studio, Silver Springs, MD
   Makeup: Juanita Diaz
   Model: Sha-Lisa Warren
   Designer/Stylist: Montgomery Harris

4a. Day Afro
4b. Evening Afro
   Stylist: Diane Bailey with Fanta Kaba
   Makeup: Roxanna Floyd
   Model: Nina Nesbitt
   Designer: Tereze Fleetwood
   Stylist: Montgomery Harris

5. Cornrows and Senegalese Twist
    Stylist: Avion Julien of Tulani's Regal Movement,
                        Brooklyn, NY
    Makeup: Juanita Diaz
    Model: Awa Sani
    Scarf: Tina Thomas

6a. Flat Twist with Lin Twist—Front
6b. Flat Twist with Lin Twist—Side
    Stylist: Cecelia Hinds of Uzuri Braids, Washington, DC
    Makeup: Juanita Diaz
    Model: Michele Bowers

7. Flat Twist without Extension
    Stylist: Cecelia Hinds of Uzuri Braids, Washington, DC
    Makeup: Juanita Diaz
    Model: Denise Fortune

8. Geni-Locs
    Stylist: Debra Hare-Bey of Red Creative Salon,
                        Brooklyn, NY
    Makeup: Juanita Diaz
    Designer/Stylist: Montgomery Harris
    Model: Kenya

9a. Silky Twist—Front
9b. Silky Twist—Back
    Stylist: N'gone Sow of Soween Braids, Brooklyn, NY
    Makeup: Juanita Diaz
    Model: Sally Toussaint

10. Weave Highlights
    Stylist: Diane Bailey
    Makeup: Anthony Jones
    Model: Merylin
    Designer/Stylist: Montgomery Harris

11. Updo Swept Locks—Spiral Curl
    Stylist: Diane Bailey
    Makeup: Juanita Diaz
    Model: Tammie Anderson
    Designer/Stylist: Montgomery Harris

12. Diamond Casama
    Stylist: Fanta Kaba
    Makeup: Roxanna Floyd
    Model: Awa Sane
    Designer/Stylist: Montgomery Harris

13. Sunburst Locs (male) & African Kurls with Flat Twist (female)
    Stylist: Diane Bailey and Tonika Outerbridge
    Makeup: Juanita Diaz
    Models: Johnna Lister and Matthew Dick
    Designer/Stylist: Montgomery Harris

14. Nubian Coils
     Stylist: Fanta Kaba
     Makeup: Susan Reed
     Model: Jean Noel

15. Silky Wrap
     Stylist: Susan Hale of African Hair Design
     Makeup: Anthony Jones
     Model: Kayan Williams
     Designer/Stylist: Montgomery Harris

16. Goddess Braids & Wrap
     Stylist: Cecelia Hinds
     Makeup: Anthony Jones
     Model: Michele Bowers

17. Nubian Coils with Nu Loc
     Stylist: Diane Bailey
     Makeup: Diane Bailey
     Model: Tonika Outerbridge

18. Stages of Locks
     Stylist: Diane Bailey and Fanta Kaba
     Makeup: Susan Reed
     Models: Soneni Smith, Sheila Johnson, Jean Noel

19a. Cornrow Braids and Singles—Front
19b. Cornrow Braids and Singles—Back
     Stylist: Diane Bailey and Kirl Alexander
     Makeup: Diane Bailey
     Model: Nicole Jorge

20. Cornrow and Casama Braids
     Stylist: Kirl Alexander
     Makeup: Diane Bailey
     Model: Fanta Kaba

21a. Pixie Braid—Front
21b. Pixie Braid—Side
     Stylist: Fanta Kaba and Diane Bailey
     Makeup: Anthony Jones
     Model: Gregg

22. Braid Royale
     Stylist: Fanta Kaba and Diane Bailey
     Makeup: Roxanna Floyd
     Model: Awa Sane
     Designer/Stylist: Montgomery Harris

23. Afro
     Stylist: Diane Bailey
     Makeup: Anthony Jones
     Model: Judy Alanna

PREFACE

I would like to give thanks to my grandmothers: Ethel, Francis, Nell and Irene for planting the seeds and nurturing my soul. Through their inspiration, life work and strong faith, I was able to flourish and grow into a re-emerged woman. They all taught me the value of community and giving back. In this book, I hope to share with the community of braiding artists and those aspiring to be natural hair care braiders/stylists, the unique and ancestral tradition of braiding.

I want to personally acknowledge the founding sisters of the International Braiders Network trade association who are visionaries and gave unconditional support in our purpose to define this new industry— Tulani Kinard, Katherine Jones, Crystal Bailes, Debra Hare-Bey, Amazon Smiley, Cecelia Hinds. Especially to Tulani, she had the tenacity and vision to petition for the New York State Braiding License. I also want to acknowledge all of my colleagues who have helped to create this industry, and who gave their technical support and time to make this book happen. Esmeralda Simmons, for her leadership and counsel that guided the enactment of the New York State Braiding License, which I believe will institutionalize and standardize natural hair care and braiding as a viable profession.

I wish to extend my special appreciation to an excellent editor and writer, Soneni Smith, who worked in concert with my vision and made me look deep into my experiences to bring forth this text. Thanks for her endless support and friendship. To Sheila Johnson, a personal friend, who forced me to see my excellence. Her unlimited energy and talent as a research library scientist proved to be an exceptional resource for this project. To Mamadou Chinyelu, for her insightful contribution in writing the history chapter of this book. Mr. Chinyelu is a historian and author of *Sons of the Prophets: 9 Inspirational Stories About African Men and Boys in the Land of Captivity* and *Debunking the Bell Curve and Scientific Racism.*

Thea Santos and Susan Bishop are lifelong sisters and lifelong friends, they have both been a lifeline for me on so many levels that the lines between our professional and personal lives are blurred. Thea has been my most faithful friend, who talks to me without words. She allowed me to experiment on her hair when I was only 10 years old. We have enjoyed good times growing into our womanhood and motherhood together. Susan kept me grounded in the business of running a hair salon and was always there to remind me of who I am. Whenever I felt challenged or defeated, Susan never let me wallow in self pity. I believe this book is a tribute to her talent as one my first braiding students and a solid friend. Though I taught Loren Baxter, a dear friend, the professional art of braiding, I can only hope that I guided her as well as she has guided me emotionally and spiritually.

To my "daughter" and sister friend, "Ka," who was born and raised on the continent of Africa and wound up in the United States and, by fate, found her way to my salon, Tendrils, in Brooklyn, NY, while I was teaching her, she was teaching me. Language barriers and cultural gulfs never defeated us. Looking back over the past 10 years, I can only believe that we were destined by the creator to be together and bring forth this African tradition.

The publisher would like to thank the following professionals who reviewed this book: Adio Akil-I, Bronx, NY; Catherine Jones, Media, PA; Amazon Smiley, Chicago, IL; and Victoria Wurdinger, Brooklyn, NY.

ACKNOWLEDGEMENTS

This book could not have been written without the unselfish support of many. I gratefully acknowledge the following individuals who contributed their time, knowledge, writings, and life experiences.

Katherine Jones, The International Braiders Network, Media, PA

Amazon Smiley, Amazon Braids, Chicago, IL

Victoria Wurdginer, freelance writer, NY, NY

Annu Prestonia, Khamit Kinks, Brooklyn, NY and Atlanta, GA

Marion Council, Designer Braids, Brooklyn, NY

Tereze Fleetwood, Phe-Zula Collection, NY, NY

Montgomery Harris, Montgomery, NY, a special thanks for creating clothing that reflects our soul's heritage

Tina Thomas, Diva Creations, Staten Island, NY

Avion Juliene, Tulani's Regal Movement, Brooklyn, NY

Adio Kas I, Praises Products, Brooklyn, NY

Tonika Outerbridge, Tendrils, Brooklyn, NY

Denise Fortune, Tendrils, Brooklyn, NY

Preston Phillips, graphic designer, Brooklyn, NY

Jaka Ray, personal chef/food specialist, Brooklyn, NY

Marshall Sohne, property management agent, Brooklyn, NY

Ona Osirio-Maat, Ona the locksmyth, Brooklyn, NY

Marion Williams, Deva by Marion Williams, unique jewelry

N'gone Sow, Soween Braids, Brooklyn, NY

Susan Hale, independent braider and designer, Brooklyn, NY

Cecilia Hinds, Uzuri Braids, Washington, DC

Susan Bishop, Jaka Studio, Riverdale, MD

Fanta Kaba, Tendrils, Brooklyn, NY

Celestine Lee, Celestine Collections, Queens, NY

Roxanna Floyd, a special thanks for your time and unique artistry, NY, NY

Neteb Ali and Fangymi Ali, Trade Beads, Brooklyn, NY

Juanita Diaz, makeup artist

Anthony Jones, makeup artist

Jeff Naeemah, Locks N Chops, NY, NY

DEDICATION

To my daughter, Kai Charisse Jackman, who can make me laugh when there are tears in my eyes, and whom I hope I can inspire to find happiness and balance. To my parents, Evelyn, Jack and Bernard for giving me choices, support and love, I hope you glow with pride. To all my clients, the braiders and natural stylists of today and those yet to come—"To thine own self be true."

INTRODUCTION

WHAT IS A PROFESSIONAL BRAIDER?

The chapter titled "The Client and You" will give you a detailed definition of what the naturalist's or braid stylist's responsibilities are to the client. The International Braiders Network (IBN) offers the following titles that will help define the hierarchy of training and skills within this growing industry.

Braid Technician

Entry level; an assistant or apprentice in the specialty of braiding. The braid technician is in the process of acquiring the various braiding techniques. This person has limited knowledge but is continuing their training.

Braid Stylist

One who has been trained and has adequate technical skills for braiding styles. The braid stylist is knowledgeable in hair loss, scalp disorders, health/sanitation, proper hair tension, and interpersonal skills; he or she understands the holistic relationship between the client and the stylist.

Braid Designer

One who is proficient and highly skilled in the art form of braiding; has more than just the technical skills; can incorporate skills into advanced techniques, creating and developing new styles. The braid designer has advanced knowledge of hair loss, scalp disorders, health/sanitation, and proper hair tension, and is one who is well versed in client/stylist relations and interpersonal communication satisfaction.

Master Braider

One who has a technical, artistic, historical, and intellectual authority of the industry of braiding and natural hair care. The master braider is proficient in creating, designing, and teaching various braid styles; can demonstrate principal skills in a minimum of ten to fifteen techniques; is a chief authority in hair loss, scalp disorder, health/sanitation, proper hair tension, and client/stylist holistic relations and interpersonal communications. Usually, the master braider has at least ten years of professional experience and several (at least two) years of teaching or training experience.

CURLS, KINKS AND COILS: WORKING WITH TEXTURE

If people knew how to work with their curly, kinky, or coiled hair, it wouldn't be necessary to spend hordes of money on products and haircuts to mask or smooth away these natural hair textures. There would be no such thing as "good" hair or "bad" hair. This natural hair care and braiding book focuses on professional techniques, herbal products, and traditional braiding, locking, and twisting hairstyles that create an aesthetic look for all hair textures. Many of these styles are cultural in origin, as they are derived from traditional African braiding designs that date back to ancient dynasties. As a professional cosmetologist, braid designer, salon owner, and an advisor to the New York State Division of Licensing, I would like to share my twenty years of experience in the hair care industry—and a deep seated need to impart information that will help stylists understand the differences in hair in a positive light—in this text, I wanted to define what is *beautiful* for naturally textured hair. I call it redefining "cultural aesthetics" through natural hair care. This is an effort to incorporate cultural standards of beauty generally unrecognized by the beauty enhancement industry, and to remove negative messages that demean African hair types in particular.

Most commercial products on the market are advertised to "rid" your hair of the frizzies, to "eliminate" kinky, tangly hair, and to control "unruly," "overcurly" hair. Straighteners are aimed at consumers who want "bone straight" or "smooth," silky hair. These advertising terms seem to imply that textured hair is problem hair, especially for people of color.

The beauty enhancement industry is biased against textured hair. An enormous amount of money is spent encouraging consumers to conform to a smooth and silky hair culture. The industry subscribes to the general philosophy that "hair is hair." This refers to the notion that all hair is alike and that the ultimate goal or preferred condition of hair is straight. This is a European standard of beauty that totally ignores the varying degrees of texture, curl, or wave formations and, of course, the grooming and styling differences that are necessary to work with textured hair.

Because of my experience with textured hair, I was asked by a law firm to consult and give expert testimony on the merits of an electric hair curling system for Asian women. I was required to test the product on Asian hair and record the results. During this case, I tested the product on eight Japanese women. Two had naturally curly hair. One, in particular, had a distinct tight curl uncharacteristic of Asian hair. This was a revelation to me. In all my years in the industry, Asian hair has been associated with being "bone straight." Further, I discovered in my interview with the woman that her curly hair was a family trait. She hated it. She and her father were scorned, and their hair was considered "inferior" simply because of its texture. The fact remains that textured hair goes beyond racial and ethnic boundaries. The wave and coil pattern of African hair is not exclusive to African people. Other ethnic groups have similar wave and coil patterns in varying degrees.

While developing this manual, I invited master braid stylists who are proficient in particular techniques to submit their work and share with readers how culturally aesthetic natural hair can be. They produced braid styles for high fashion, casual, and career looks. The "cultural aesthetic" standard appreciates the beauty in other ethnic communities, which are inspired by their beliefs, customs, behavior, and technical skills. What is significant about African braiding and natural hair care is that it can be appreciated by all people as a cultural art form. Braid styles are now being integrated into the contemporary beauty enhancement industry's diverse approach to hair care. The other benefit of developing a cultural aesthetic is that when men and women are comfortable with wearing styles that are culturally relevant to them, they are affirmed and empowered.

NATURAL HAIR IS VIRGIN HAIR

Virgin hair has not been chemically altered in texture, color, or volume. Virgin hair is not pressed or altered by excessive heat, electric curling, or other thermal services. Any treatment that destroys or breaks down the natural coil pattern of the hair strand (meaning that the hair will not return to its original coiled pattern) denatures the hair. If the hair has been altered chemically, it requires six months to a year to grow into its natural state.

It is important to note that as states begin to adopt "Natural Hair Care" licenses, the rules and regulations governing the license may allow services that contradict what natural hair should represent. For example, the New York State Natural Hair Care license allows natural hair to be thermally altered, but restricts stylists from coloring natural hair. In New York, you must have a certified cosmetologist license to chemically color hair. Many people become confused and think that pressing is a natural service simply because it does not involve chemicals.

Structurally and biochemically, all hair types are similar. The industry divides hair types into three ethnic groupings: European, Asian, and African. Biochemically, hair is the same for all racial groups and, structurally, they are similar. All hair, regardless of texture, has the same basic parts: a root, a bulb, a follicle, a hair shaft, and a cortex, among other structural components. In textured hair, however, these basic components take on a different formation and therefore it differs in its physical appearance (refer to Chapter 5 "How Hair Types and Structures Differ"). The degree of texture is directly related to the development and shape of the follicle. Textured hair or coiled hair is not a "deformity" or misfortune as advertisers would have you believe. Textured hair is not "problem" hair. Textured hair is manageable.

MARKET AND INDUSTRY INFLUENCES

For African-Americans, straightening the hair is a "hair conforming" behavior that has existed since slavery (refer to Chapter 1 "History Overview"). This behavior has led to a systematized pattern of hair abuse and texture denial, as well as created a large profit on straightening products in the hair care industry. Statistics indicate that more than $4.5 billion dollars a year is spent on hair grooming products. These numbers indicate just how intensely people groom their hair. Paula Begoun, author of *Don't Go Shopping For Hair Care Products Without Me*, explains, "To facilitate and *atone* for the damage caused by the straightening process, the ethnic hair-care market is overflowing with product choices. The statistics are nothing less than boggling." She adds, "African-Americans buy more than 37% of all hair care products even though they comprise only 12% of the population, and wash their hair, on average, no more than once every seven to fourteen days (compared to Caucasians and Asians, who wash their hair an average of four to five times a week)."

The African-American community is spending great sums of money to conform to a "straight and silky" hair culture. They spend even more on conditioners and treatments to maintain chemically damaged hair. With all the buying power in the African-American community, and the sophistication of hair care products on the market, hair damage and hair abuse in the African-American community is nearly epidemic. The industry has forced people of color to deny their natural texture, to choose styles and treatments that are damaging and, in some cases, have proven harmful to their health. There are class action suits filed against certain companies that claimed they could straighten hair "naturally" without chemicals. For some, these so-called "natural perms" have caused hair loss maladies and various scalp irritations. (See Chapter 6 "Hair and Scalp Disorders and Diseases".)

If the industry maintains that "hair is hair," why is it that large marketing divisions of hair care companies distinguish between ethnic hair care product lines and mainstream hair products? Walk into any drug store and you will find that hair products for the African-American and Latino consumer are segregated from the general consumer hair products. If shampoo is shampoo and "hair is hair," then all shampoos should be on the same shelf. The industry has placed new emphasis on marketing ethnic specialty products even for braid styles. There are numerous books, magazines, and videos addressing the needs of textured hair. Why? Because textured hair is "other" to the industry. I believe African hair *is* different—wonderfully different. Not since the Afro in the 1960s has there been such a re-emergence of wearing naturally textured hair among African-Americans and Latino people. However, unlike the 60s, natural hair and braid sculpted styles are not necessarily political statements. Men and women who choose to wear their hair naturally are making a statement about themselves. It is more than a cosmetic change or fashion statement, but an expression of self. They are saying "I am." They are breaking the myths that once surrounded textured hair. They are more culturally exposed, and generally health conscientious. They are secure in their being with or without straight hair. This newly defined self also empowers and frees people to be true to themselves. It is an inner awakening that broadens a person's self-image. Through self-image, African-Americans as well as other ethnic groups are defining what is culturally aesthetic to their community.

From this textbook, I look forward to seeing students and professionals alike understand and embrace the basic traditional approach to hair care that is nurturing and affirming. You will understand the holistic approach to hair care and the harmonic balance between healthy hair (your outer beauty) and spiritual health (your inner beauty). You will empower your clients to be free of chemical and thermal processing, and to show appreciation to their virgin hair with gentle, wholesome, and nurturing services.

ABOUT THE AUTHOR

As a natural hair care specialist, I too have experienced an inner awakening and total self-acceptance of my hair. It was liberating. I am now actively working to empower other stylists, industry professionals, and consumers. There is an African proverb that says "The world is a mirror: show yourself in it and it will reflect your image." I must have always known this, in my own special way. I saw my hair as a creative outlet at the age of nine, experimenting with myself by cutting my hair. As it grew back, I stopped at any reflection of myself—water puddles, car windows, or storefronts—to comb and groom my hair and my bangs. At the age of 21, and after graduating from Hunter College, no one was surprised when I entered beauty school—that's what they called it then.

In beauty school, I became frustrated by the bias and limited approach to hair care. They focused on the care and treatment of straight hair. There were no classes that dealt with "virgin" hair—hair that was not chemically straightened. Once I began wearing a small Afro, I was ostracized and questioned as to why I wouldn't "perm" my hair. I was thrilled when I met a fellow female student who could braid hair with extensions. I had never seen anything like it, and that was twenty years ago. She taught me, and I practiced on myself. We learned from each other, and we taught ourselves intricate braid designs and styles.

When I became a promotional model at Bloomingdale's, I was approached by a customer who asked me to "fix" her hair. I was wearing large single plaits with diagonal parts at the time. About that time braid styles were just beginning to be worn by celebrities such as Cecily Tyson and Roberta Flack. The matriarch of braiding at that time was Black Rose, known to everyone in the Black hair industry. Ellen Levar, another pioneer, was the featured braid stylist for *Essence* magazine. I started braiding at home, like many still do today. I was part of the cottage industry. From time to time, I worked in "uptown" Harlem hair salons and at Hair Fashions East with well-known stylist George Buckner.

I became involved in the natural hair movement when, in 1987, I was invited to the second annual convention in Chicago by the National Braiders Guild (NBG). The NBG was founded by Hiddekel Burk, a Chicago braider. The weekend convention attracted nearly 300 professionals from around the country. But the concept for the NBG convention was actually conceived in 1982, when the Smithsonian Institute in Washington, D.C. hosted an African Arts exhibit that featured traditional African hair braiding. It was the first time that a major institution of this magnitude recognized braiding as an art form. At the same time, Pam Ferrell and her husband Taalib-Den Uqdah were pioneering the development of a braiding license in Washington, D.C.

By 1988, NBG had widened its scope and hosted a Natural Hair and Braiding conference. That year I held a workshop on locking hair and Ademola Mandella instructed a barbers workshop. The natural hair concept was becoming more inclusive. To meet the needs of this expanding movement, the International Braiders Network (IBN) was founded in 1992 in New York City. That same year, Tulani Kinard, one of IBN's founders, Amedola Mandella and Esmeralda Simmons, director of the Center for Law and Social Justice in New York, began lobbying and drafting the first Natural Hair Care license. The license was adopted on July 5, 1994 and provided a one year grandfather clause for licensing existing braiders and anyone who could show proficiency in the art.

As president and a co-founder of IBN, our trade association has been instrumental in developing and promoting natural hair care throughout the nation. We recognized early that cosmetology law in the United States had not been updated since the 1930s. We came together in order to establish professional standards, procedures and training for natural hair care stylists and braiders.

IBN goals:

1. *To establish a worldwide network of professional braiders, lockticians, and natural hair care specialists.*

2. *To promote the cultural, historical, and technical aspects of braiding, locking, and natural hair care.*

3. *To establish an educational foundation that addresses the needs of natural hair care specialists within the beauty enhancement industry.*

NOTES

The terms naturalist, natural hair care specialist, braid stylist, *and* braid designer *may be used interchangeably in this book. Although they have different levels of skills and training, the author refers to them inclusively because of the industry's basic natural hair care ideology.*

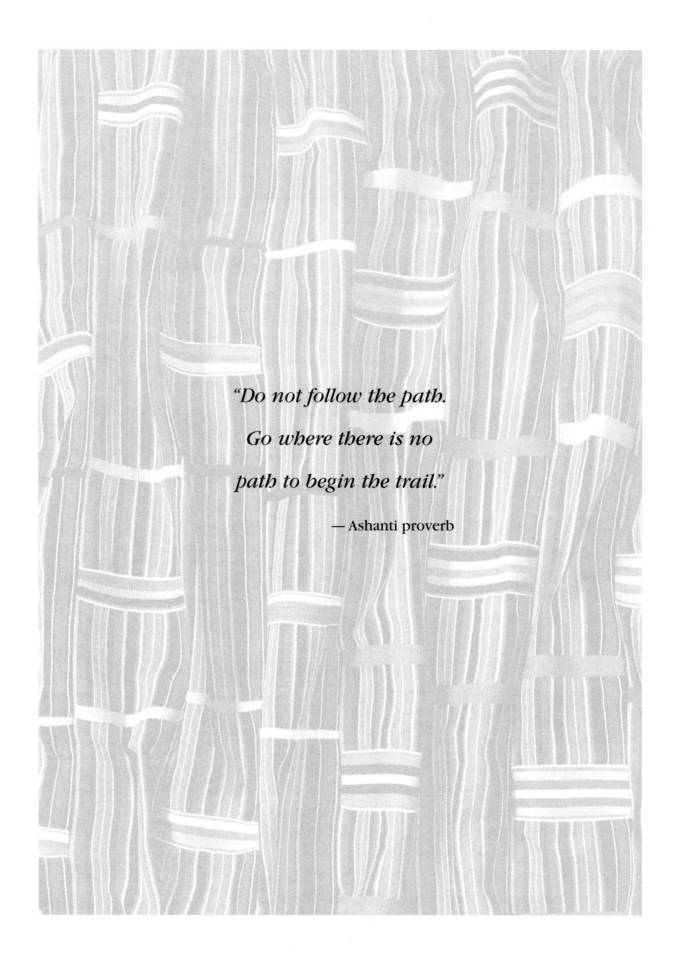

"Do not follow the path.

Go where there is no

path to begin the trail."

— Ashanti proverb

CHAPTER

1

History Overview

by Mamadou Chinyelu

KNOWLEDGE BOX

In this chapter you will learn:

1

The ancient origins of hair braiding

2

Traditional African braid styles

3

What certain braid styles communicate

4

The African-American hair experience

INTRODUCTION

Hairstyles in the African tradition have often reflected the legal, social and political status of African people. For many people today, hair-styles are more a matter of personal choice than a political statement. This brief overview of the African hair braiding tradition and the styles that people of color have chosen to wear over the years demonstrates how trends and social structure in American society have influenced self-image.

ANCIENT ORIGINS

Hair braiding has been the most enduring hairstyle in the African tradition, including cornrows, box braids and plaits.

Hair braiding has been the most enduring hairstyle in the African tradition, including cornrows, box braids and plaits.

Although there is no substantial body of literature on the history of hair braiding, the art of braiding was not lost. Records of African hair braiding can be found in the ancient stone sculptures and other engraven images that withstood the test of time. Through these images the tradition of hair braiding, unique to Africans, can be traced to the very threshold of civilization.

One of the earliest recorded images of hair braiding can be traced to Saqqara, on the tip of the Nile Delta, near Memphis, the capital of the First Dynasty founded by Pharaoh Manes. Saqqara is the burial site of predynastic kings and queens. From this location was found a piece of the tomb of Akhethoptep, now in possession of the Brooklyn Museum, in New York, that shows the government official not only holding his symbol of authority, a staff and scepter, but also wearing braids. This plate is dated to the late Third Dynasty at about 2630-2540 B.C. Another object at the Brooklyn Museum that exhibits a man wearing braided hair is found in the late Fourth Dynasty sculpted head of a Courtier, an attendant in the pharaoh's court. Braided hair is also evident in the image of Seshemnofer II, one of the last kings of the Fourth Dynasty. The original home for this piece of art depicting the head Seshemnofer II was Giza, the site of the pyramids built by Pharaoh Khufu. It can now be found in Alabama, at the Birmingham Museum of Art.

Hair braiding, like other prominent cultural practices, was maintained wherever Africans traveled. Such was the case with Africans who journeyed to pre-Columbian Mexico (about 800-400 B.C.). You can find a unique style of hair braiding on the colossal pre-Columbian stone sculpted head of an African man.[1] Another example of hair braiding, is found on a Sixth Century clay pouring vessel from the Congo region that shows an African woman wearing a braid style fashioned vertically and wrapped with beads.[2] Toward the modern era, a 16th Century artifact, a bronze plaque, depicts the King of Benin's hair braided in an intricate multi-tiered fashion, as is the hair of some of his attendants.

BRAID STYLES

Historically, there has always been a variety of hair braiding styles. The styles in the African tradition were not for beautification alone. In many instances, different styles symbolized a person's stature in an African society. Hair braiding was a non-verbal form of communication. Certain styles told you certain information about a person. For example, married women wore different styles than maidens. "The most elaborate hairstyles have always been the privilege of married women. Even today, in Fouta Djalon, Guinea, Fulani women wear a style—an architectural triumph in itself—in which the hair is molded into shapes like huge butterfly wings. Further east, the Kanuri women of Lake Chad, part of the former kingdom of Bornu, wear impressive plaits of hair running from the forehead to the nape of the neck," according to Angela Fisher, author of *Africa Adorned*.

Hair braiding was a non-verbal form of communication. Certain styles told you certain information about a person.

"Married women of the Songhai Empire (10th to 16th Century of the Christian Era) wore a braid style that featured a circular woolen disc at the front," Fisher noted. Pregnant women also wore braid styles that distinguished them from other women. In ancient Egypt, pregnant women knotted "their hair behind the head in a large bun, or in numerous plaits which would then hang down at either side of the head."[3]

---

[1] Ivan Van Serima, <u>They Came Before Columbus</u>, (plate 4a), 1976.
[2] Leon E. Clark, <u>Through African Eyes, Vol. 1, The Past: Road To Independence</u>, 1988, 91.
[3] Bernard Romant, (translated by J. Smith), <u>Life In Egypt In Ancient Times</u>, 1986, 30.

Among other nations, hair braiding styles revealed the sex of the recently born child. The Rendille women of Kenya, upon giving birth to a son, wear their hair in plaits known as a "coxcomb," and the style is maintained until the son is circumcised. African braid styles have also provided information as to the age, social standing, economic status, occupation, and geographic location of the wearer. Of course, many braid styles are fashioned purely for vanity's sake. Of the Congolese women, one writer says, "A woman's beauty is judged by the manner in which her hair is dressed." In ancient Egypt, the "more coquettish" women wore fancy headbands around their braids.

Given the variety of styles, many designs were given imaginative names such as "boat of the sky, bellow of the forge, and spend the night with the one you love."[4] It should be remembered that the ancient and modern tradition of hair braiding was practiced by both men and women. Some of the more elaborate braid styles, just as today, required as many as three days to perfect.[5]

Hair braiding can be viewed as the artistic or ceremonial expression of the science of agriculture.

BRAIDING'S AGRICULTURAL ROOTS

The science of agriculture came to Africans first, and it is one of their many gifts to civilization. In tilling soil, farmers used a hoe-like tool to make rows in the earth; they fertilized the soil and planted seeds. They pulled the weeds and waited patiently until a harvest was produced. From this perspective, hair braiding can be viewed as the artistic or ceremonial expression of the science of agriculture.

The basic techniques of hair braiding require the similar exercise, or practices, of agriculture. A comb is used to make parts in the scalp much like the hoe used by farmers. The braider often oils the scalp (as in fertilizing the soil). The root of hair is already planted. Braiders trim and groom the hair just as farmers cultivate and weed the plants. As a result, the wearer of braids often experiences longer, healthier hair (the harvest). Even the braid style called "cornrow" is a direct agricultural term. When Africans worked in cane

---

[4] Angela Fisher, <u>Africa Adorned</u>, 148-149.
[5] Ibid., 42.

fields the braid style was called "cane row." It takes little imagination to see that agriculture not only served as a model for hair braiding, but also created the leisure time that made hair braiding possible. The domestication of food production was a landmark in the history of human civilization. It allowed some families to be "released from the food hunt to other specialties: tool-making, shelter building, potting, organizing the tribe, medicine …"[6] It also created more time for adornment such as hair braiding.

HAIR LOCKING

Before moving forward on the historical timetable, let us step back to the period that predates hair braiding and agriculture (when people gathered food to eat). Africans wore a hairstyle that we know today as locks—a natural process for uncut and meshed African hair. Locks are mentioned no fewer than seven times in the Bible. (The Lord told Moses to say to the Israelites: When anyone, man or woman, makes a special vow dedicating themselves to the Lord as a Nazerite … the whole term of their vow no razor is to touch their head; they must let their hair grow in long locks until they have completed the term of their dedication; they are to keep themselves holy to the Lord.) According to the Bible, Samson, the most famous judge of the Israelites, wore seven locks, the source of his divine strength. It will be argued by some that it is presumptuous to say that references to locks in the Bible refer to African hair because the only concept of locks for many people is the childhood reference to Goldie Locks, a European fairy tale character. There are, however, Europeans whose hair appears to be locked the same as African locks.

Hair locking is as natural to the African race as other common physical traits.

Another fallacy about hair locking is that Rastafarianism, a spiritual approach to life that originated in Jamaica, gave birth to hair locking. This is not true, and not everyone with locks is a "Rasta." Hair locking is as natural to the African race as other common physical traits. According to Adio Ras I, a New York locktician and manufacturer of Praises, a line of natural hair care products, who has spent years researching the origin of locks, "African priests, prophets and scientists grew their hair long as a testament of their

---

[6] Lester Brooks, <u>Great Civilizations of Ancient Africa</u>, 1971, 17.

separation from the ways of the world and toward the ways of the creator." Hair locking today is a standard natural hair care practice. Specialists in this area are "lockticians," who are trained to groom and sculpt locks.

THE EFFECTS OF AFRICAN SLAVE TRADE

Africans existed as a self-determined, self-defined and self-reliant people. This existence was brutally interrupted in the 15th Century by what is known as the African slave trade. It was a time when African people were uprooted and dispersed throughout the world, particularly to the western hemisphere. For the first 400 years, Africans were victims of chattel slavery.

Due to a lack of hair tools and lowered self-esteem, Africans produced hairstyles distinctly different from the pre-slave trade.

During the physical enslavement period, Africans had no rights. They were valued for their labor and their ability to breed more chattel. Working from sun up to sun down left no time and little reason for adornment. The once regal hairstyles degenerated to shapeless, ungroomed hair. Without their traditional tools to groom African hair, the slaves often covered and wrapped their hair with cloths. In a testament to African resilience, however, a basic plaiting style was commonly employed in an effort to maintain a sense of pride and African tradition.

Because of this period of physical bondage and humiliation, the lack of hair tools and lowered self-esteem, African slaves produced hairstyles distinctly different from the pre-slave trade.

PRESS AND CURL

Freed but not quite liberated, Africans had the leisure to give personal grooming the attention befitting all. However during the centuries of physical slavery, most African people were coerced into believing that European cultural norms were superior to African cultural norms. Hence, when Africans regained the leisure to groom themselves, they did so in the European image, trying to emulate their standard of beauty and making tightly curled African hair straight.

They would apply heat with hot knives or forks, or sandwich their hair between hot metal to elongate it. The process became somewhat perfected when, in 1905, Madame C.J. Walker introduced "a hot iron for straightening the hair of Negro women." With the hot iron, the Black beauty culture industry was born. Another leading pioneer of the beauty culture industry was Annie Turnbo-Malone, who developed beauty schools and hair products. The industry opened new avenues, outside of domestic work, for African-American women to enter the work force. Many women sold specialty beauty and hair care products door to door.

The struggle to end slavery was in the recent past. The new struggle was to be accepted as American. At the turn of the century, fewer Africans in America thought about returning to Africa. Many African-Americans were eager to belong and be respected. The "press and curl" quickly became the hairstyle that respectable African-American women wore. The perfected "press and curl" became the industry standard and remained so throughout the 1960s. Even today, many hair salons continue to provide the traditional "press and curl" service.

The struggle to end slavery was in the recent past. The new struggle was to be accepted as American.

PERMS AND THE MODERN WOMAN

The press and curl gave African women in America the look they wanted, but it proved not to be a long lasting hairstyle. In the African-American home, press and curl was the Saturday ritual. Women would spend half the day "getting their hair done" for either the party on Saturday night or for church on Sunday morning. The pressed styles had to be maintained until the next press and curl by either rolling the hair in strips of brown paper bags, with store-bought curlers or by tieing scarfs around their heads to keep the hair flat and straight. Some women would restrict activities, such as swimming and sports, to keep their hair from "turning back" or getting wet, and in order to maintain the fresh pressed look as long as possible. Within days, however, the pressed hair would lose its straight or hot curl look, become bushy from the humidity or moisture, and return to its naturally textured African hair.

Soon another straightening process known as **perms** (for permanent) or **relaxers** was developed to ease tight, curly hair. This chemical straightening was also adapted for men and commonly referred to as the **process** or **conk**.

Perms and conks were lye-based chemical straighteners. They used strong, harsh chemicals that often burned the scalp and, in some cases, created permanent hair loss. "Konkaleen" was the most popular brand among men, leaving the hair bone straight. In the 1950s, the leading manufacture and pioneer of chemical relaxers was George Johnson, founder of Johnson Products. Posner was another major Black-owned hair products company that produced chemical relaxers.

These straighteners boosted the Black hair care industry tremendously and gave African hair the European look that many desired for social acceptability. In addition, it was long-lasting and durable. To maintain the look, perms required repeated touch-ups as new curly growth appeared. It required more visits to the beautician and became costly to maintain. The "permed" look soon became synonymous with affluent African people who were better educated and often employed in professional job situations.

The Afro returned African grooming tools, such as wood-carved pics and rakes, back to the Black hair-care industry.

THE AFRO

Chemical innovations and straight hair could not, however, mask the turbulent years of racial violence, Jim Crow laws, and segregation that African-Americans had suffered. No straightener could ease the frustration nor stop the revolution of new thinking on the rise that ultimately propelled the Civil Rights Era and the Black Power Movement.

Young African-Americans rejected the European look and embraced African styles which became known as the **Afro**, **Bush**, or **Natural**. The Afro was a controversial style. It was considered a hostile act to wear an Afro, and myths that the Afro style would cause lice and premature baldness abounded. The style endured and grew in popularity as a sign of African beauty and self-esteem, particularly during the 1960s. The significance of the Afro, according to hair historians, is that it returned African grooming tools, such as beautiful wood-carved pics and rakes, and natural hair oils back to the Black hair-care industry—fine-toothed European combs and harsh shampoos were insufficient to maintain a well-coifed Afro.

At the height of the Afro's popularity in the 1970s, the blown-out Afro style quickly became a fashion statement (a hair trend) and less of a political statement. The Afro was worn by African-Americans and whites alike. It was the "Age of Aquarius." The production of *Hair* was a raging success on Broadway. People felt free to "just be." The Afro was embraced by the popular culture and many ethnic groups. The style was worn by celebrities and leading sports figures. Brightly colored Afro wigs were common on the disco dance floors and the popular television dance show *Soultrain.*

THE JHERI CURL

Named after its inventor, Jheri Redding, the **Jheri Curl** sent a clear message to forget about Africa—just "relax." By 1977, Willie Morrow created the popular **California Curl**. The Jheri Curl and the California Curl offered style options to African-American men and women. These cold-wave relaxers maintained the curly textured look of an Afro, but simulated shiny, soft, glossy, tamed curls. The cold-wave curls appeared less "threatening" than the Afro of the 60s and less flamboyant than the blown-out Afro of the 70s.

The cold-wave process involved chemicals to straighten the hair, and then more acid-based chemicals to create a wave.

This cold-wave process involved heavy chemicals to straighten the hair, and then more acid-based chemicals to create a wave. To maintain the shiny look, a sticky, drippy moisturizing spray had to be applied daily along with an activator solution that kept the chemically straight hair curled. Some men and women fashioned plastic caps and bags on their heads to retain the activator/moisturizer on the hair for longer periods of time. Without the moisturizer the chemically treated hair would dry out and break.

THE NATURAL '90S

If there is a direct link to natural hair care, the economy, political climate and cultural awareness, then the stock market crash of 1987, the rise in unemployment, global awareness, the expanded information highway, and the end of apartheid has greatly influenced how people of color choose to wear their hair.

Still looking for simple solutions and with a greater sense of cultural pride, more African-Americans are wearing their hair naturally textured and braided and it is becoming widely accepted. Men and women are more conscious of their health in general and are looking for alternatives to chemical treatments. As the society grows more complex, some people are going back to what is culturally familiar.

Though the Jheri Curl and other chemically straightened hairstyles for African hair have not disappeared, natural hairstyles and braids have returned to prominence on a level that has not been seen in hundreds of years in the African-American community.

Intricate African braid styles and weaving patterns have been resurrected by professional stylists and talented people who have perfected African braiding and restored it to its proper cultural art form. The demand for such styles is growing as Africans in America are frequently traveling to Africa. They are decorating their homes in African motif. They are reading more about African history and expressing an interest in African affairs. These expressions of self-love are an attempt at a powerful emergence of self-healing.

Intricate African braid styles and weaves have been resurrected and restored to their proper cultural art form.

The various hairstyles worn by African people today are braiding, wrapping, twisting, locking, and natural hair cuts. These techniques serve as a telling metaphor for the history of African people, ancient and modern, on the continent of Africa and throughout the world—that the more you struggle, the more inclined you are to return to your "roots."

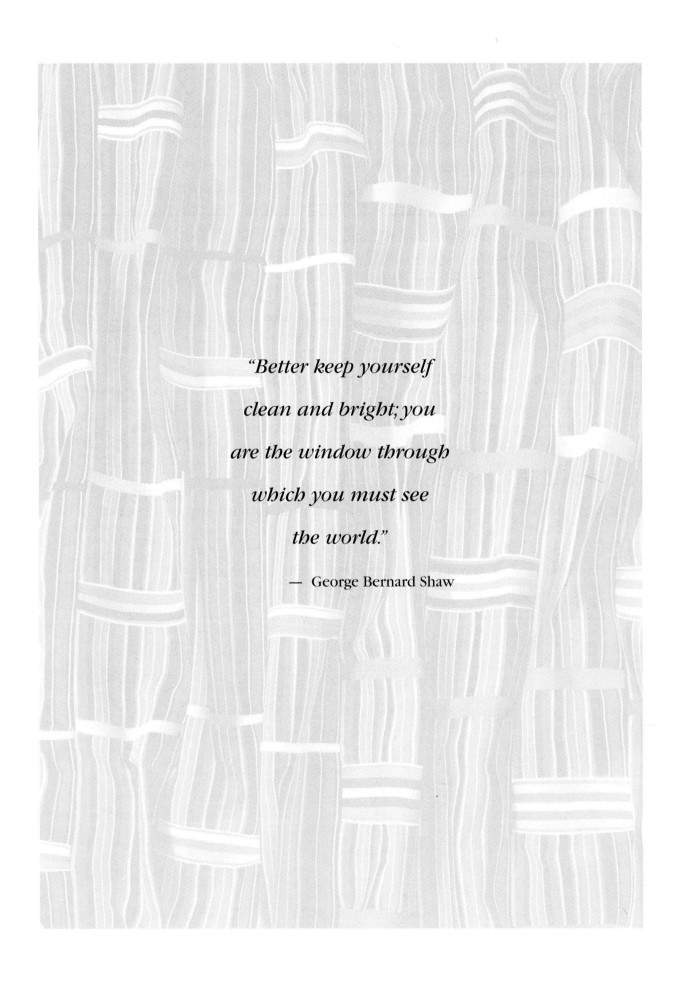

"Better keep yourself

clean and bright; you

are the window through

which you must see

the world."

— George Bernard Shaw

CHAPTER

2

Bacteriology/Sanitation & Prevention Control

KNOWLEDGE BOX

In this chapter you will learn:

1

Definition and types of bacteria

2

How bacteria grows and reproduces

3

The relationship of bacteria and the spread of disease

4

Prevention and infection control

5

Standard sanitation practices

6

How to use antiseptics, disinfectants, and detergents

INTRODUCTION

Bacteriology, sterilization, and sanitation are subjects of practical importance to you as a stylist, because they have a direct bearing on your well-being as well as on your client's welfare. To protect individual and public health, every stylist should know when, why, and how to use good sterilization and sanitation practices.

In order to understand the importance of sanitation and sterilization, a basic understanding of how bacteria affect our daily lives is most helpful.

PREVENTION AND INFECTION CONTROL STANDARDS OF HEALTH AND SANITATION

Bacteriology is the science that deals with the study of microorganisms called bacteria. These are minute, one-celled vegetable microorganisms found nearly everywhere. Bacteria, also known as germs, are especially numerous in dust, dirt, garbage, and diseased tissues. They can exist nearly anywhere including skin, water, air, clothing, and beneath nails.

Listed below are the two types of bacteria:

Nonpathogenic—decomposes refuse and improves soil fertility. Example: *saprophytes live on dead matter and do not produce disease.*

Pathogenic—harmful, produce disease when they invade plant or animal tissue. Example: *Parasites require living matter for growth.*

CLASSIFICATIONS OF PATHOGENIC BACTERIA

Bacteria have distinct shapes that help to identify them.

Pathogenic bacteria are classified as follows:

1. *Cocci are round-shaped organisms that appear singly or in the following groups:*

   a. *Staphylococci: pus-forming organisms that grow in bunches or clusters. They cause abscesses, pustules, and boils.*

   b. *Streptococci: pus-forming organisms that grow in chains. They cause infections such as strep throat.*

   c. *Diplococci: grow in pairs and cause pneumonia.*

2. *Bacilli are short rod-shaped organisms. They are the most common bacteria and produce diseases such as tetanus (lockjaw), influenza, typhoid fever, tuberculosis, and diphtheria.*

3. *Spirilla are curved or corkscrew-shaped organisms. They are subdivided into several groups. Of chief importance to us is the treponema pallida, which causes syphilis.*

MOVEMENT OF BACTERIA

Cocci rarely show active motility. They are transmitted on the air, in dust, or in the substance in which they settle. Bacilli and spirilla are both motile and use hairlike projections, known as flagella or cilia, to move about. A whiplike motion of these hairs propels bacteria about in liquid.

How Bacteria Grows and Reproduces

Bacteria manufacture their own food from the surrounding environment, give off waste products, and grow and reproduce.

The two distinct phases in their life cycle are:
<u>*Active (vegetative stage)*</u>—*Bacteria grow and reproduce; they*

multiply in warm, dark places with sufficient food. Once they reach their largest size, they divide into two cells, also known as mitosis.

Inactive (spore-forming stage)— Spores may form on certain bacteria to withstand unfavorable conditions (famine and dryness). Can be blown about and are not harmed while in this stage. When conditions are favorable, they change into the active phase.

BACTERIAL INFECTIONS

There can be no infection without the presence of pathogenic bacteria. An infection occurs when the body is unable to cope with the bacteria and their harmful toxins. A local infection is indicated by a boil or pimple that contains pus. The presence of pus is a sign of infection. Bacteria, waste matter, decayed tissue, body cells, and living and dead blood cells are all found in pus. Staphylococci are the most common pus-forming bacteria. A general infection results when the bloodstream carries the bacteria and their toxins to all parts of the body, as in syphilis.

A disease becomes contagious or communicable when it spreads from one person to another by contact. Some of the more common contagious diseases that prevent a stylist from working are tuberculosis, common cold, ringworm, scabies, head lice, and virus infections.

The chief sources of contagion are unclean hands and implements, open sores, pus, mouth and nose discharges, and the common use of drinking cups and towels. Uncovered coughing or sneezing and spitting in public also spread germs.

A disease results when bacteria is carried throughout the body. It becomes communicable (contagious) when it spreads from one person to another.

Some common contagious diseases are:

- *tuberculosis*
- *common cold*
- *ringworm*
- *scabies*
- *head lice*
- *virus infections*

The main sources for spreading diseases are:

- *unclean hands and implements*
- *open sores*
- *pus*
- *mouth and nose discharges*
- *common use of silverware, cups, or towels*
- *uncovered coughing or sneezing*
- *spitting*

Infections can be prevented and controlled through personal hygiene and public sanitation.

Pathogenic bacteria can enter the body through:

1. *A break in the skin, as with a cut, pimple, or scratch*
2. *The mouth, through breathing or swallowing air or food*
3. *The nose*
4. *The eyes or ears*

The body fights infection by means of:

1. *Unbroken skin (the body's first line of defense)*
2. *Body secretions (such as perspiration and digestive juices)*
3. *White blood cells (which destroy bacteria)*
4. *Antitoxins (counteract the toxins produced by the bacteria)*

OTHER INFECTIOUS AGENTS

Filterable viruses are living organisms so small that they can pass through the pores of a porcelain filter. They cause the common cold and other respiratory and gastrointestinal infections.

Parasites are organisms that live on other organisms without giving anything in return.

Plant parasites or fungi, such as molds, mildews, and yeasts, can produce contagious diseases, such as ringworm and favus, a skin disease of the scalp.

Animal parasites are responsible for contagious diseases. For example, the itch mite burrows under the skin, causing scabies, and infection of the scalp by lice is called pediculosis.

Contagious diseases caused by parasites should never be treated in a beauty school or salon. Clients should be referred to a physician.

IMMUNITY

Immunity is the ability of the body to destroy bacteria that have gained entrance, and thus to resist infection. Immunity against disease can be natural or acquired and is a sign of good health. Natural immunity means natural resistance to disease. It is partly inherited and partly developed through hygienic living. Acquired immunity is something the body develops after it has overcome a disease, or through inoculation.

It is good business to have a safe and harmonious working environment. It is also the law.

A human disease carrier is a person who is personally immune to a disease yet can transmit germs to other people. Typhoid fever and diphtheria can be transmitted in this matter.

Bacteria can be destroyed by disinfectants and by intense heat achieved by boiling, steaming, baking, or burning, and ultraviolet rays.

GOOD HABITS

The primary difference between the professional and non-professional braid stylist is the high standards of health and sanitation maintained in the salon. An orderly and clean hair salon offers a harmonious and safe environment for the client. It is paramount that the natural hair care specialist's central focus in the salon is to provide an environment free from dirt, dust, oils, infectious diseases, and germs. It is the braid stylist's responsiblity to clients and co-workers to ensure their safety.

Providing a harmonious and safe environment is more than just weekly cleaning. It is the continuous practice of preventive procedures, the expedient care of tools and surfaces, and personal hygiene that minimizes and controls the spread of infection.

If a client or co-worker becomes seriously ill because of inadequate care of tools or an unsafe work environment, the salon owner can be held liable and irreparable damage can be done to the business. If clients lose confidence in the safety of the braiding at a salon, they will not return for further services. As an entrepreneur it is good business to have a safe and harmonious working environment. It is also the law.

State and federal regulations require that certain preventive measures against the spread of infectious disease and germs be taken or the salon operator's business can be shut down. Each state has specific regulations that address the responsibilities of the salon owner as well as a renter of a salon booth. These regulations are standardized health and sanitary codes which hair care specialists, braiders, lockticians, and barbers must comply with.

If you are already licensed, your training covered the state and federal regulations. Keep them handy and refer to them often. Be sure to check for changes and updates.

If you do not have your license, you should get access to the regulations to make sure you are in compliance.

Everything in the salon has a working surface: the tables, counters, chairs, floors, shelves, mirrors, tools, and implements. All surfaces, especially tool surfaces, must be kept free from contaminants such as dirt, oils, debris, and micro-pathogens. By removing these disease-causing substances, you are decontaminating your salon. Decontamination of tools and surfaces is maintained on three levels: sanitation, disinfection, and sterilization.

Decontamination of tools and surfaces is maintained on three levels: sanitation, disinfection, and sterilization.

Sterilization is the highest form of decontamination. The process of sterilization actually kills germs including the most resistant form of bacterial spores. Bacterial spores are very resistant to many disinfectants and can be "up to 10,000 times more resistant to disinfectant than when it is in its active, growing form."[1] To sterilize tools and implements, a sterilizing chamber such as a steam autoclave is used. The steam autoclave (often seen in dentists' offices, doctors' offices, or nail salons) works like a pressure cook-

---

[1] Chesky, Sheldon R., Cristina, Isabel, Rosenberg, Richard, Playing It Safe, Milady's Guide to Decontamination, Sterilization and Personal Protection, Albany, NY: Milady Publishing, 1994, 35.

er. It uses high heat and steamed pressure to kill all living organisms. Unless the braid stylist uses tools that puncture or break the skin, sterilization is unnecessary and can be impractical. It is unrealistic to believe that you can sterilize the entire work environment and tools without using hazardous hot fumes. So, the most practical methods of decontaminating the salon are sanitation and disinfection.

SANITATION AND DISINFECTION

To sanitize is to reduce the germs with the use of soaps and detergents.

The most well-designed salon can lose its attractiveness if it is not routinely sanitized. To sanitize is to reduce the germs in the working environment with the use of soaps and detergents. Daily cleaning may be sufficient in a small salon (serving one to two clients per day). However, medium to large (five or more clients) salons must be sanitized and kept orderly several times each day. It is important that each braid stylist be responsible for their immediate working areas as well as common areas, such as the shampoo sinks, hair drying areas, bathrooms, and eating areas. Disinfection controls and kills specific microorganisms on tools and other implements.

Tools must be cleaned before disinfecting. This means that tools must be scrubbed with soap and water before placing them into a disinfection solution. There are several different professional soaps and detergents that specifically address the removal of germs from tools. Some commercial home products—bleach and pine-oil cleaners—can be used to remove dirt and grease from surfaces of floors, chairs, counters, shelves, door handles, and telephones. However, these products can be expensive as well as ineffective and damaging to the tools.

The following is a general guide to keeping the salon environment harmonious, safe, and clean.

1. All glass shelves and mirrors should be cleaned daily.

2. Windows should be routinely cleaned.

3. Garbage receptacles must be covered and emptied daily. (Garbage is a very opportunistic habitat for bacteria, germs, rodents and insects. In high-traffic salons, remove trash several times each day.)

4. *Floors should be kept free of debris and unused working materials.*

   > *When working with hair extensions, material often falls on the floor. Hair must not accumulate or obstruct passageways in the work space.*

   > *Remove all extension material around the chairs and floors, as well as any material that falls into the chairs.*

   > *Wipe surfaces clean and remove all debris before seating a new client.*

5. *Mop floors with detergents daily and after any spills (to prevent injuries from slips and falls). Also, vacuum carpets and doormats. Keep floors in good condition.*

6. *Remove dust, debris, and oil from all surfaces including dryer hoods, ceiling corners, walls, shelves, and baseboards.*

7. *Air conditioner filters, fans, and ventilators must be cleaned regularly. If you use a humidifier or steam vaporizer to prevent mold growth, clean the water reservoir daily with a vinegar solution.*

8. *Plumbing fixtures for wash sinks, toilets, and shampoo sinks must be maintained and kept in good condition. These, too, are inspected for compliance with state and local codes.*

9. *Bathrooms must be cleaned daily or more often for high traffic salons.*

10. *Bathrooms should always be equipped with an ample supply of paper towels, toilet tissue, and a pump-type antiseptic liquid soap. Commercial bar soaps do not have antibacterial properties. Bar soaps sit in a dish and often carry bacteria, transmitting germs to others (also known as cross-contamination).*

11. *Bathroom handles should be wiped or sprayed with a disinfectant regularly.*

12. *After using the restroom and between client services, hands must be scrubbed with an antiseptic liquid soap for several minutes. Waterless hand cleansers are also available.*

13. *Sinks and neck rests must be sanitized after every service. Sinks should have hot and cold running water.*

14. *Smoking is prohibited in the work area of the salon. Separate areas should be designated for smoking and eating.*

15. Eating and drinking must never be done while servicing a client. Take a break between braiding sessions for relaxing and eating.

16. Cooking is prohibited in a working salon. Food preparation should be done in a separate room with adequate ventilation of exhaust fumes.

17. Any living quarters must be separate from the work area.

18. Refrigerated foods must be kept separate from salon products to prevent ingesting hair preparations. Some natural oils and herbal solutions should be kept in a cool place; however, never store them with food.

19. Braid stylists must wear clean, ironed clothing without tears and holes, or uniforms and smocks to protect from dirt and hair clipping debris.

20. Stylist must wear shoes. Shoes should have the appropriate support for long-standing braid services. Cross-infection of fungi such as athlete's foot can be avoided by wearing shoes.

21. Each client must always be given clean, freshly laundered towels.

22. Cloth or paper towels must never be shared. All wet or soiled towels must be removed from the sinks and countertops and placed in hampers.

23. Combs, brushes, clips, and disposable caps must never be shared.

24. Tools or implements that fall on the floor should never be used until scrubbed with soap and water and then submerged in an Environmental Protection Agency (EPA) grade disinfectant solution before reusing.

25. All tools must be soaked in an approved disinfectant solution for at least ten minutes or more, then rinsed, dried, and placed in a clean drawer or covered container.

26. Client capes or covering must not ever touch bare skin. A towel or paper neck strip must be used before draping a client.

27. Client capes must be laundered regularly.

28. Combs, clips, curlers, and pins should not be placed in stylist's mouth or pockets.

29. All containers should be properly labeled.

   Outside of containers must be cleaned after every use, tightly sealed, and properly stored.

> ⧫ Inside of disinfectant containers must be cleaned regularly. Cloudy solution is a sign to discard and replace with a fresh solution to avoid cross-contamination.

30. Pets are prohibited in the salon, except those animals that assist the visually impaired or physically challenged.

31. Young children should not be allowed to run around the salon so that injuries, such as burns or ingestion of hair products can be prevented. They should not be allowed to play with hair tools.

32. Open flames, gas burners, or lit candles are prohibited. To singe extension braids, small cigarette lighters can be used effectively and safely. Hold lighters away from the client's face.

33. Electric teapots can create different finishes on braids. To avoid accidents, drape the client with several towels and a water repellant shampoo cape.

34. Avoid cross-infection by not touching your face, hair, mouth, eyes, or arms when servicing a client.

35. Wear plastic gloves whenever possible. When removing braids or weaves, gloves will protect the stylist's hands from dirt and debris.

36. To avoid contamination, never reuse synthetic or human hair. Briefly worn human hair wigs, hair pieces, and weaved hair may be reused if shampooed, conditioned, and rinsed thoroughly (smell is a good test for freshness).

37. Always keep in compliance with individual state and federal laws and regulations to avoid fines and reprimands.

The primary function of OSHA is to regulate, monitor, and ensure employee safety from toxic materials.

Salons and schools are subject to inspection by the Occupational Safety and Health Administration (OSHA) and state boards of beauty enhancement. OSHA focuses its safety and health concerns on the work environment and employee protection. The primary function of OSHA is to regulate, monitor, and ensure employee safety from toxic materials used in the work area. The braid stylist is vulnerable to daily exposure to bacteria and infection. Although natural hair care specialists do not use chemicals to alter hair textures, other chemicals in the salon such as antiseptics, cleansers, disinfectants, shampoos, and conditioners may be used. OSHA also sets standards for mixing, storing, and disposing of chemicals and hazardous products. It is the stylist's responsibility to be aware of product contents in order to protect themselves and their clients.

HOW TO USE ANTISEPTICS, DISINFECTANTS, AND DETERGENTS

The most effective way to use cleansing agents is to read the labels. Read all instructions carefully before handling disinfectants. Effective disinfectants must be registered and approved by the federal Environmental Protection Agency (EPA) and state departments of environmental protection. Disinfectants used for tool "reprocessing" must have an EPA designation as a **hospital-grade** disinfectant or germicide. Germicides actually kill and destroy dangerous bacteria.

It is a federal law that all disinfectants provide important information such as:

- *a list of active ingredients*
- *directions on effective and proper usage*
- *safety measures and precautions*
- *a Material Safety Data Sheet (MSDS)—an information sheet that provides content and active ingredients, dangers, combustion levels, and storage requirements. MSDS must be kept for review and inspection. This is a federal requirement*

Disinfectant Safety

Always use caution when using disinfectants. Be sure to wear gloves and safety glasses while mixing or using. Never pour alcohol, quats, phenols, or any disinfectant over your hands. Never place any product in an unmarked bottle.

Other Surfaces

There are many surfaces in the salon which require disinfection. Some commonly used tools are:

- *combs*
- *brushes*
- *scissors*
- *razors*
- *nippers*
- *electrodes*

Surfaces to consider sanitizing are:

- *table or counter tops*
- *telephone receivers*
- *door knobs*
- *cabinet handles*
- *mirrors*
- *cash registers*

Other tools to remember to sanitize include:

- *mixing utensils*
- *pins*
- *clips*
- *curlers*
- *hair dryers*
- *chairs*
- *fans and/or humidifiers*

Always remember: sanitation removes and kills <u>some</u> germs, disinfection kills and controls <u>most</u> germs, and sterilization destroys <u>all</u> germs.

NOTES

ANTISEPTICS

Antiseptics are sanitizers that are safe to use on the skin, scalp, and hair. They are weaker than disinfectants; however, antiseptics can reduce and kill bacteria. Liquid antiseptic soaps are excellent for cleaning visible dirt and oils and removing bacteria. For minor cuts and burns, antiseptic creams, gels, or liquids should be used to protect from infection. Examples include witch hazel, peroxide, or commercial first-aid ointments. When using commercial antiseptic creams or gels, look for the active ingredients. Such creams as Bacitracin® or Neonycen® can prevent infection and aid the healing process.

After applying any ointments or liquids to clean cuts or burns, cover with a bandage. First-aid kits are available with various types of antiseptics. Always follow the package directions.

Antiseptics are sanitizers that are safe to use on the skin, scalp, and hair.

NATURAL ANTISEPTICS

Every natural hair care salon should also have first-aid staples on hand. Aloe vera gel and tea tree oil should always be on the shelf. Aloe vera gel can be found bottled or in its most natural state—the plant. The plant is a native of Africa and the Mediterranean region. It has been used for hundreds of years in these areas. The aloe plant is characterized by its long, tapered, thick green leaves. When the leaves are broken, a light emulsive sap exudes and can be applied externally to cuts and burns. The gel soothes itching and burning directly after it is applied. It aids in the regeneration of new tissue when scarring and normal pigmentation has been affected. Adding benzoin tincture to aloe vera can make an antiseptic solution that prevents blistering.

Tea tree oil is known as the "medicine kit in a bottle." This oil is a native of Australia. Tea tree oil is a clear aromatic oil that will increase the healing process. It soothes insect bites, herpes sores, cuts, burns, and fungal infections. This antiseptic oil will increase the process of healing burns or cuts because it escalates skin regeneration. Normal pigmentation loss can return if used consistently. Tea tree oil is also effective on itchy scalps and dandruff.

DISINFECTANTS

Each state regulates and registers disinfectants, sanitizing, and sterilant agents. The state boards of cosmetology and licensing, the state boards of public health, and OSHA all set the standards for proficiency to protect the braid stylist in the industry. The EPA sets the high standards for manufacturers of products that claim to kill germs, fungi, or viruses. The EPA registration number is given to products that have the highest level of germicidal, fungicidal, or virucidal effectiveness. The EPA number is your best insurance that the product will do all that it says it will do.

Read the MSDS and the label. The label gives instructions on how to use the product, the active ingredients it contains, and how to store and dispose of the product. Read several times before using to get the best results (Fig 2.1).

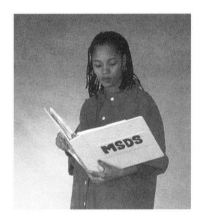

Figure 2.1 Read your Material Safety Data Sheets (MSDS).

Household disinfectants will not kill the various bacteria you will be exposed to when braiding hair. Household disinfectants are the lowest level for killing germs and can be very expensive. The EPA hospital-grade disinfectant is specifically produced to work efficiently in a working environment and to kill organisms.

Do not take short cuts or use less expensive products. Always use the best products to protect yourself. The stylist is more at risk than the client, because you are exposed for a longer period of time and to more people. Keeping a safe and harmonious environment is your responsibility and will affect your salon's reputation.

VIRUSES AND INFECTIONS IN THE SALON

In a salon setting, stylists may be exposed to the following virus and fungal infections: common colds, influenza, measles, chicken pox, mumps, herpes I and II, hepatitis A and B, and the human immunodeficiency virus (HIV).

Common colds are transmitted by hand-to-face, physical contact. Hepatitis B and HIV can be transmitted by blood and body fluid cross-contamination.

Fungal infections such as nail fungus, ringworm, and athlete's foot are easily spread in an unkempt salon.

Hepatitis A and B Viral Infections

Hepatitis A and B are viral diseases that attack the liver. The liver is a vital organ that produces chemicals that aid the human body in metabolizing foods and drugs. The most apparent symptom of this disease is a yellowing of the skin and the whites of the eye. This is called jaundice.

Hepatitis A is contracted through the digestive system. Contamination is usually directly related to raw or improperly cooked food and dirty utensils. Contaminated tools and implements can spread this infectious virus through direct contact with saliva and other bodily fluids.

Hepatitis B is a more serious infection because it has greater health complications. It is often fatal. Transmission occurs through direct contact with blood, saliva, semen, and other bodily fluids.

Disinfectants are the commercial and professional substances that are used to kill germs.

DISINFECTANTS FOR TOOLS AND SALON

After sanitizing tools or surfaces with soaps and detergents, pathogens and bacteria continue to live. Sanitation alone does not stop the spread of infectious germs. Disinfection is the next level of decontamination. Disinfectants are the commercial and professional substances that are used to kill germs.

For the best results, it is recommended to use an EPA approved disinfectant to ensure that the product is effective. Look for the EPA registration number. These hospital-grade disinfectants kill most bacteria and viruses (including HIV). Germicides are excellent products to use in the salon and will exceed the minimum state requirements for safety.

All disinfectants must have directions on how to prepare or use the product safely and list active ingredients on the MSDS. It is very important to properly use disinfectants. A disinfectant will not work effectively if hair, scalp debris, and oil contaminate the solution.

Reprocessing standards when using disinfectants are as follows:

1. After each service, scalp debris and hair can be removed by raking through the implement. Pull loose hair, debris, creams, and gels to the surface of the implement. Rinse well to avoid solution contamination.

2. Implements can then be scrubbed with warm water and soap detergent.

3. Rinse thoroughly and dry with a clean towel.

4. Tools are immersed in a hospital-grade disinfectant solution. Implements must soak in the disinfectant for at least ten minutes.

5. After removing implements from the solution, rinse with warm water, dry, and store separately with other clean tools.

6. Electric clipper heads, razors, scissors, and needles for weaves can be immersed in a hospital-grade disinfectant. Soak for ten minutes. Rinse and dry. A spray disinfectant can be used before each use in the client's view.

7. Liquid disinfectant containers—glass or plastic—should be cleaned and solutions changed daily, according to manufacturer's instructions.

8. Disinfectant solutions should be stored and maintained to avoid contamination. Clean and monitor areas where solutions are stored. Protect labels by wiping sealed bottles with a clean cloth so that instructions and other important information remains legible (Fig 2.2).

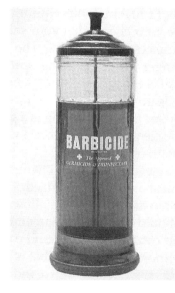

Figure 2.2 Implements should be thoroughly cleaned before soaking to avoid contaminating the disinfecting solution.

TYPES OF HOSPITAL-GRADE DISINFECTANTS

Alcohol

Ethyl alcohol (ethanol or grain alcohol) is the most effective strength for disinfecting tools and has a 70% or greater alcohol content.

Isopropyl alcohol (rubbing alcohol) is the most effective strength for disinfecting and must be a 99% solution.

The braid stylist should have both alcohols available for use in the salon although they are not specifically designed to disinfect professional tools. The EPA recognizes them as an adequate disinfectant that will stop the spread of bacteria. However, there are some disadvantages when using alcohols. They are extremely flammable, evaporate quickly, and are slow-acting, less effective disinfectants. Alcohols corrode tools and cause sharp edges to become dull. The vapor formed upon evaporation can cause headaches and nausea in high concentrations or after prolonged exposure.

HIV & PERSONAL PROTECTION

Treat every client with a high standard for their safety and your protection from disease.

Aquired Immune Deficiency Syndrome (AIDS) is a fatal disease caused by the human immunodeficiency virus (HIV). This virus destroys the body's defenses against disease and infection. People infected with HIV may show no symptoms for years (in some cases ten to fifteen years). HIV in itself does not kill the victim. The infections from common microbes or germs break down the body because the body's defenses have been destroyed. It can not fight or heal from infection. At the present time, there is no cure for HIV.

As a braid stylist you can be at risk to contract HIV. However, the risk is very low and HIV is difficult to spread in a hair salon setting. Still precautions are necessary because everyone is at risk if exposed to blood, open cuts, mucous membranes or other body fluids (semen) infected with HIV. The risk is created if, when servicing a client with the virus, the client is accidently cut, nicked, or scraped and the stylist has open wounds. If the client and stylist interact and infected blood gets into an open wound, there is a risk that the HIV virus could be spread.

However low the risk, concern requires that universal precautions be taken. This means that you treat every client with a high standard for their safety and your protection from disease. You cannot look at a person and determine if he or she is HIV infected. There are many infectious diseases and taking precautions with all clients lessens your chances for exposure.

COMMON SENSE PROTECTION

There are several simple steps you can take that will greatly reduce your chances of infection.

1. *Avoid touching any open cuts or sores your client may have (usually in the scalp area).*

2. *Wear disposable latex gloves when blotting blood, or when putting antiseptics on the cut. <u>Never use bare hands.</u>*

3. *Immediately after removing gloves, wash and scrub hands with antibacterial liquid soap.*

4. *Place all tools used in a germicidal disinfectant and follow directions.*

5. *Disinfect counters, chairs, towels, and capes regularly after servicing clients.*

6. *Discard towels or cotton used to wipe bloodied areas or to cover bare skin (usually the neck area).*

7. *Tie plastic trash bags and place apart from the work area.*

8. *Evaluate if client looks jaundiced. If you feel she may be jaundiced, recommend a doctor.*

9. *Clean and disinfect work area after every client.*

10. *To avoid exposure, a Hepatitis B vaccine is available to prevent infection.*

TYPES OF DISINFECTANTS

There are several types of disinfectants you can use effectively in your salon to minimize the risk of contamination.

1. *Barbicide—for cleaning tools and hair implements.*

2. *Household bleach—for cleaning bathroom sinks, towels, and floors after sanitizing (washing with detergents).*

3. *Iodine-based compounds—for cleaning floors, walls, chairs, and countertops.*

4. *Quaternary ammonium compounds (quats)—very safe and fast acting; for tools, tables, and counter tops.*

5. *Phenolic disinfectants (phenols)—used to disinfect implements, may cause skin irritation.*

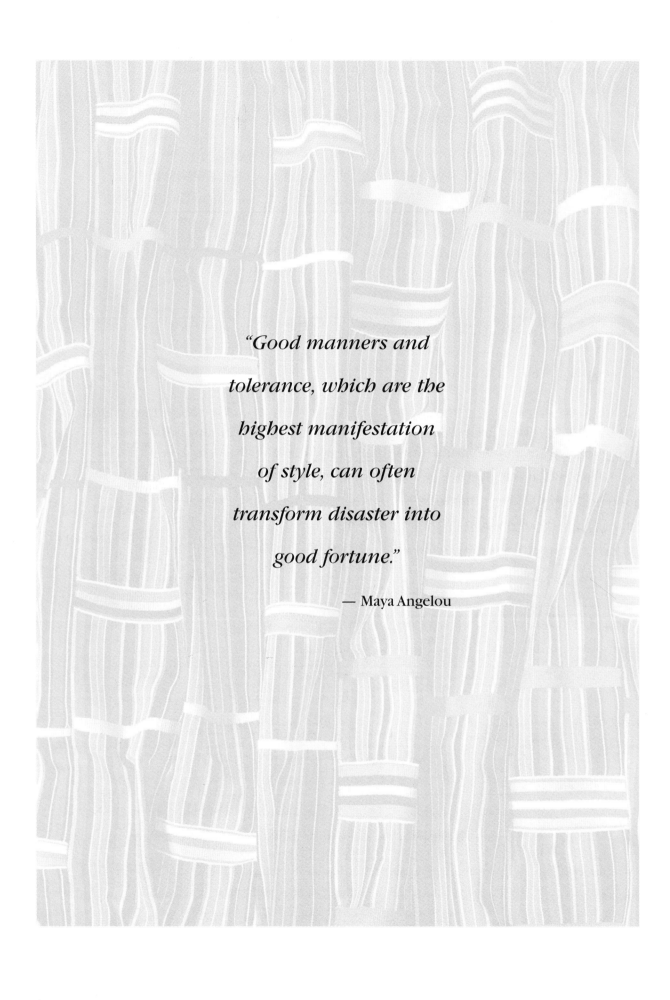

"Good manners and tolerance, which are the highest manifestation of style, can often transform disaster into good fortune."

— Maya Angelou

CHAPTER

3

The Client and You

INTRODUCTION

There are distinctive attributes in the relationship between the natural hair care specialist and the client. In general, the beauty industry focuses primarily on efficiency and services, rather than the total well-being of the client. But in the field of natural hair care, the stylist must be able to recognize the interrelationship between the client's hair, body, emotional, and physical environment in order to achieve the best results and have a satisfied customer.

In the natural hair care industry, the stylist is first faced with having to focus on improving the client's self-image. To redefine your clients' self-image means to change or enhance your clients' mental picture of themselves. This involves improving their outer image and their mental picture so that both reflect a whole, self-accepting and beautiful person. As a natural hair care specialist, one opens the boundaries and opens minds that beauty is inherent in all people regardless of race and hair texture.

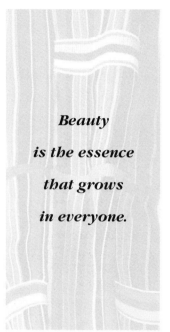

Beauty

is the essence

that grows

in everyone.

Beauty starts from within. It is the essence that grows in everyone. It is more than a reflection in a mirror. To be beautiful is to find the innate harmony between one's emotional self (spiritual) and one's physical image. This harmony can be nurtured by the stylist, for example, by grooming the hair without altering the texture, braiding, conditioning, locking, cutting, and weaving. Together the client and stylist can re-establish a balance of self-respect for the client's natural hair texture.

Many of your clients will have little or no adult history of wearing their hair in its naturally textured state. For many clients, childhood memories have left only negative impressions. Improper tools, poor grooming skills, and negative social images have scarred many clients. For African-American clients, in particular, many may still consider their hair **kinky** or too nappy. When they come to the salon, they may be choosing for the very first time to wear their hair braided publicly. It is not unusual, in the beginning, for the client to be apprehensive about wearing their natural hair or hair extensions.

A stylist cannot remove all the negative experiences, but by redefining what is culturally aesthetic—that appearance which is in accordance with your sense of ethnic customs or beliefs—and by providing current grooming techniques and styles, the stylist can educate and correct the client with discovery of her inner beauty.

Redefining words like nappy or kinky is the beginning of educating the client. These words are descriptive aids to define texture; they are similar to terms like straight, wavy, or curly. Hair having a very tight curl pattern can be described as kinky or nappy. As professionals, these terms are not definitive to hair texture, but are lay terms to help clients describe their hair texture. Hair that has curl patterns can be described in terms of its spiral or coil configuration. A coil is a very tight curl. As the hair lengthens, the patterns resemble a spiral or a series of loops. There are several different types of coil patterns (which will be discussed later). Stylists who can describe their clients' hair with a different perspective—using new and old terms to describe hair textures—help their clients to overcome the negative views of their hair or self-image.

THE HOLISTIC APPROACH

A holistic approach integrates all factors into a program designed for the client's complete well-being.

A holistic approach to nurturing the client is one of the unique aspects of this rewarding industry. The natural hair care specialist focuses on the physical, psychological, and the emotional needs of the client. A holistic approach integrates all these factors into a program designed for the client's complete well-being. The stylist must be able to understand the external and internal stresses that affect the client's total well-being. With this approach to natural hair care, the stylist views the beauty and health of the client as being equally important. A natural hair care stylist must never endanger the client's hair in order to create a fashionable style. The natural hair care specialist's view is that it is better to prevent than to cure. Avoiding harsh chemicals, abusive tools, and excessive styling practices are preventative measures in keeping hair healthy.

The naturalist is acutely aware that an attractive client is a healthy client. The whole person is equal to the sum of his/her parts and, as a result, a healthy client will have healthy hair. Your "inner" health is reflected in your hair. Good nutrition, exercise to maintain good circulation, and a peaceful or stress-free emotional state of mind are the components to healthy hair. We do not live in a vacuum. Therefore, our environment affects our hair. Poor air and water quality, lack of vitamin D (from the sun), and stressful work or home environments are some of the external pressures that affect the hair and cause hair loss.

With the holistic approach, the stylist is aware of these interrelated factors and is capable of educating clients, raising client consciousness, and reconnecting them to their natural hair. And so with the natural hair care salon, the stylist offers a more quiet, relaxed, spa-like environment that includes soothing music, proper lighting, ample ventilation, and inspiring or invigorating colors.

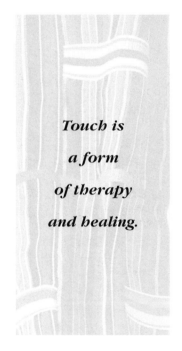

Touch is

a form

of therapy

and healing.

BUILDING TRUST THROUGH TOUCH

Being touched and having the ability to touch is a vital human need. The natural hair care professional is basically licensed to touch.

As infants we need to be held or stroked. This physical motion of stroking communicates reassurance and comfort. It has been well documented that touch is a form of therapy and healing. Some medical authorities agree that the "therapeutic touch may work simply because it raises the patient's spirits and as a result, the bodily defenses. As holistic medicine teaches, anything that makes you feel better can also influence your recovery." [1]

As a professional natural hair care stylist, ones hands are "healing" tools. Shampooing, massaging, braiding, or locking should be calming, lulling, and gentle. The client should always be in a relaxed state. Some braiding styles are more soothing than others. In such cases where the braiding may be more stressful, the client should be informed prior to the service. The touch used in providing any natural or braiding service is not only a relaxing

---

[1] Scoleri, Donal W. and Lasoncy, Lewis, MD, The New Psy-Cosmetologist, *Salon Today*, 1998, 8.

technique but can also be a stimulating technique. A soft but firm deliberate touch is what will create the style. When braiding, the stylist's fingertips—*not* the entire weight of the hand—are used to execute the technique.

The stylist's touch is also therapeutic and nurturing to the client. The repeated massaging and touch releases stress and begins to break down the client's inhibitions. The client becomes more open, spiritually and emotionally. There can now be an exchange between the two people. A healing energy is transmitted. Studies have been done at the University of Maryland Medical School by Dr. James Lynch, a specialist in psychosomatic medicine, which reports that "petting animals has a beneficial effect on people's cardiovascular systems; it also increases their resistance to infection…even people in deep comas often register improved heart rate and brain waves when their hands are held by doctors, nurses, or family members."[2] This study demonstrates that there is a real connection between touch, feeling good, and healing.

The naturalist's goal, then, is to reassure and comfort the client so that he or she makes the right styling choices. In addition, the stylist must also realize that healthy hair is more than what is used topically on the head. Healthy hair is the result of a healthy body and mind. For example, in our hectic lives, stress can be a major factor in certain hair loss problems. So it is imperative that in a natural hair care salon, the specialist offers a more quiet, relaxed, spa-like environment. This comfort level will begin to set the tone for the client/stylist relationship.

Healthy hair is the result of a healthy body and mind.

Some clients look to the stylist to motivate, nurture, and respond to their day-to-day life stories. It is at this special moment that a more personal bonding between the client and stylist takes place.

The relationship between the stylist and client can be compared with a doctor/patient relationship. In that sense, natural hair care specialists become more than artists or hair designers. They become what typically is nicknamed in the industry as "hair doctors."

[2] Scoleri, Donald W. and Lasoncy, Lewis, MD, The New Psy-Cosmetologist, *Salon Today*, 1998, 15-16.

> ***The client/stylist intimate contact generally begins with these three procedures:***
>
> *1. A relaxing, rhythmic shampoo that is also a stress-releasing scalp massage. It removes more than dirt and oil—it also removes the client's inhibitions.*
>
> *2. Hot oil conditioning treatments that range from stimulating and refreshing to slow and relaxing, creating a soothing experience.*
>
> *3. Herbal rinse or deep conditioning, fortifying hair and "rinsing" the client.*

Sharing and personal exchange leads to an extended-family-like environment within the salon.

These three procedures often allow clients to expose themselves, their flaws, and their concerns. As the client becomes more vulnerable to the specialist, the stylist often begins to see a different side of the client's personality. This relationship intensifies as the client reveals his or her imperfections. The interaction builds to a level of total acceptance as the client's fears and self-doubts are lowered. This acceptance also allows the client to feel safe and not judged. Acceptance and a wonderful shampoo/conditioning experience deepens the relationship between the stylist and the client; trust starts to flourish.

Within a period of one year, a stylist may service each client at least six to as many as twenty-five times. During that time, a specialist is privy to many of the client's life-changing experiences such as births, deaths, graduations, divorces, and weddings. This sharing and personal exchange leads to an extended-family-like environment within the salon. The trust factor that evolves over time creates a bond and a sense of security that positions the stylist as the client's confidant.

MAINTAINING A PROFESSIONAL ATTITUDE

The key to a professional relationship with your clients is learning to develop effective communications skills and maintaining a level of professionalism without alienating the client.

The various forms of communications are:

- Attitude
- Tone of voice
- Body language
- Manner of dress
- Personal grooming

There are basically three styles of communication: passive, aggressive, and assertive.

Passive—Underreacts to situations: never takes responsibility for mistakes; lets others make decisions for them; usually has soft voice; has low self-esteem.

Aggressive—Overreacts to situations; takes too much responsibility for others; gives unasked-for advice; makes decisions for other people; criticizes (constructive or otherwise); has a loud voice; is pushy and/or bossy; always knows better than everyone else.

Assertive—Effective in a positive way; reacts to situations appropriately; willing to listen; is open; has high self-esteem; shares observations and respects others' points of view; presents a good attitude; stays balanced; controls emotion and does not let emotion control them.

In business, as in life, a person whose communication style is more assertive is generally more successful than those people who are too passive or aggressive.

There are basically three styles of communication: passive, aggressive, and assertive.

Techniques for good communication:

1. *Listen to what is being said and what is not said.*
2. *Always try to mirror the client, matching verbal and nonverbal communication (body language).*
3. *Give feedback, and answer questions and comments.*
4. *Try to respond to the client's needs.*

Using these communication techniques, the client and stylist become more comfortable in one another's presence. It will also assist the stylist in meeting the client's expectations.

To the client, the stylist is immediately viewed as a professional simply because the client sees a professional as one who earns his/her livelihood by performing specific skills and services. Therefore, at all times the stylist must project a proper image and positive attitude, be of good character, and adhere to simple moral codes of ethics.

CODE OF ETHICAL STANDARDS

Ethical conduct will create honest, stress-free relationships with those around you.

In the beauty enhancement industry, each state has a set of standards of conduct that all stylists must follow. Ethics are a set of standards, moral judgements, and compliances determined by the state board of cosmetology. They are standards of behavior which a professional hair care specialist is expected to reflect. These codes of ethics are not just rules and regulations, but are informal expectations of a professional in the industry.

As a business person, the stylist must handle transactions with many different people effectively. Co-workers, clients, repair-people, and sales distributors are the kinds of people you can come in contact with daily.

Ethical conduct will create honest, stress-free relationships with these people that will not only enhance your professional image but help operate your business profitably. Ethical conduct improves your reputation in the community and builds a client's confidence in you, so much so that your clients begin to refer others to you. Personal referrals are the best form of promotion to keep your business successful.

The following is a basic code of conduct you should practice:

1. *Always remember that the service you offer is a reflection of you. Your work is an extension of yourself.*
2. *Give everyone the best quality you can physically offer. Be capable and competent.*

3. *Avoid making offers of services you cannot efficiently provide. If a client requests a style you cannot do, do not do it.*

4. *Be honest with all people. Your reputation depends on it.*

5. *Be courteous. You will meet people from different cultures and backgrounds. Respect their feelings, religious beliefs, and customs.*

6. *Comply to all state regulations. By following them you are contributing to the health and welfare of your clients.*

7. *Maintain a safe environment not only for your clients but your co-workers too.*

8. *Sell products and services that the client needs or wants. Do not be overzealous in promoting a particular line of goods unless you truly believe in it.*

To improve and maintain a professional image, stylists should always look to upgrade their skills and work on self improvement. Whenever the opportunity presents itself, a stylist should look at improving or keeping up with the following:

- *Braiding and style techniques*
- *Industry innovations*
- *Management skills and technology*
- *Self-image*
- *Communications skills*

> *The client is looking for someone to guide him/her through the transition of "going natural."*

PREPARING CLIENTS FOR THE NATURAL HAIR CARE SERVICE

Keeping in mind that the special relationship between the client and stylist is holistic, the kinds of services a specialist provides are mostly therapeutic—not in a medical sense but in a manner that gives the salon a spa-type quality.

The average client that walks into a braiding salon generally has a history with chemically treated hair. The client is looking for someone to guide him or her through the transition of "going natural" or wearing "chemical-free" hairstyles.

For the client who has suffered any amount of hair loss or scalp damage, the naturalist or braider is particularly needed to restore, treat, and correct the abused hair.

For the client who has little or no history with chemically treated hair, the specialist can offer preventive services to aid the client. The client with natural, healthy hair is offered an array of sculpting and grooming services to maintain healthy hair.

In some cases, the natural hair care specialist and braid designer work in conjunction with a dermatologist, or assist clients with scalp disorders to treat and camouflage hair loss.

The naturalist is available to coach clients in discovering themselves without the use of chemicals, to help them abandon the social confines of what is traditionally accepted as "beautiful," and to redefine what is naturally aesthetic.

The naturalist is available to coach clients in discovering themselves without the use of chemicals.

The following is a list of basic hair care services that are essential and particular to the natural hair care specialist. The natural stylist:

- *helps clients understand and appreciate the natural beauty which is inherently their own, through historical photos and braid style books.*
- *focuses on the positive attributes of textured hair: its strength, luster, and ability to grow.*
- *helps clients see their hair's potential.*
- *redefines how clients view their hair by teaching clients to respect their hair in its natural state.*
- *builds clients' self-confidence by helping them to look good and feel good about their natural state.*
- *helps clients create a positive self-image.*
- *demonstrates and explains the internal and external factors that directly affect healthy hair.*

The naturalist or braid stylist also offers the following:

1. A specialized skill in the art of hair braiding and beauty

2. Expertise on certain braiding techniques

3. Treatment of the hair as a canvas in order to create individual styles. No two people are alike!

4. Familiarity with the latest styles and trends

5. Knowledgeable advice to provide clients with enough information so that the client can make an educated decision

6. Style options and guidance on maintaining styles

NURTURING THE CLIENT'S TOTAL WELL-BEING

After the stylist has gained the client's trust, the client respects the stylist as a professional and there is a clear understanding of what services are being provided. The final step in the client/stylist relationship is learning how to nurture the client's total well-being. Perhaps in no other field of cosmetology today is this aspect of hair care so vital to the naturalist and braid designer.

The final step in the client/stylist relationship is learning how to nurture the client's total well-being.

African braiding styles have been controversial in the work place to the extent that some salons provide legal assistance and counseling for clients determined to wear what is culturally aesthetic to them.

Intricate braiding styles and fashions can take eight to ten hours, sometimes days, to complete. They are generally not disposable hairdos that can be washed away or brushed out. With proper care a braiding pattern can last up to three months. Clients must understand that they will be living with a particular hairstyle for long periods of time. Therefore, the client must be committed to the hair design and have a positive self-image to carry it off through what can be called a "hair recovery/transitional phase." This transitional phase connotes the time and/or process in which the client's hair grows "back" significantly in length and volume. This process can take several months or up to two years depending on the damage of the hair and the desired length the client is trying to obtain.

It is not uncommon for a stylist to refer clients to another stylist simply because a client is too apprehensive and not quite ready for the total natural or braided look. The last thing a stylist wishes to do is spend hours on a braiding style and have the client reject it, demanding that all the braids be removed. Not only is it time consuming for the stylist, but it could mean a loss of income for the business. Consultations, which are discussed in Chapter 4, are extremely important in determining a client's readiness—especially when the client wants the ultimate natural style: locks.

Nurturing and supporting clients are not simple matters for most hair salons. There have been clients whose jobs were in jeopardy simply because they chose to wear Africentric braiding styles to work. At the start of the client/stylist relationship, a stylist must decide what his/her level of support will be to the client.

Help the client to understand the general physical connection to having healthy hair.

Another aspect of the client's well-being is helping them understand the general physical connection to having healthy hair. This is a process of reeducation for many clients. This may require coaching on diet and nutrition and providing general health literature in the salon for the clients to read.

When working with a client, a stylist can quickly identify early signs of stress and thinning hair. This is more readily observed when the hair is natural as opposed to being chemically treated. With chemically treated hair, such problems as hair loss, thinning, and breakage can be directly related to hair products, so such problems are not often seen as stress-related hair loss. Yet, helping clients learn to cope with stress may be another way in which the stylist deals with the total well-being of the client. Once again, good communications skills will help to determine what the client's needs are.

To deal with the well-being of the client, the stylist must be prepared to do the following:

1. *Coach the client through the hair recovery/transitional phase of natural hair care.*
2. *Dispel the myths and stigmas of naturally textured hair and culturally aesthetic hair fashions.*
3. *Educate the client about health and nutrition, suggest reading materials, and provide relevant information.*
4. *Refer new clients to other clients that are successfully wearing natural and African hairstyles.*

5. *Keep an open dialogue with the client to allow them to release and discuss their concerns.*

6. *Follow up with clients, helping them to see themselves as others see them.*

Marion Council, ten-year owner of Designer Braids and Trade, Inc., of New York and Virginia, sums it up (in a telephone interview with the author) by confirming what was said earlier: "When the commitment is made to open the doors of a professional braiding or natural hair care salon, a real commitment is made to customer service and open honest communication. One's creativity will flow, unbounded, once a relationship is set."

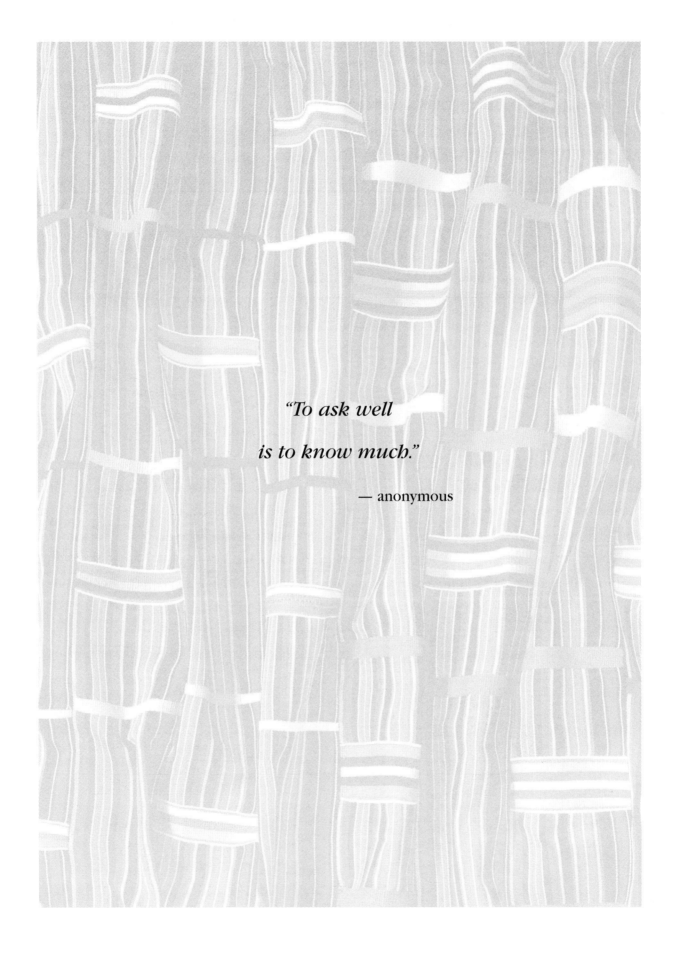

"To ask well

is to know much."

— anonymous

CHAPTER

4

The Professional Consultation

INTRODUCTION

The consultation between the new client and the naturalist is the greatest opportunity for the stylist to determine precisely what a potential client's needs are and to avoid client dissatisfaction with the end result. This is also a key step in developing a bonding relationship between the stylist and client. During the consultation, the stylist is focused on the client's hair, needs, and personal expectations while at the same time deciding whether the client can be helped or not.

No stylist in business for themselves would suggest turning customers away, but sometimes it is in the stylist's best interest to be forthright with potential clients and, if necessary, refer their business elsewhere. In the end, the stylist earns more respect and the client, if he/she decides to become a customer, will be even more satisfied with the process.

The consultation is the opportunity to determine what a client's needs are and to avoid dissatisfaction.

There is no time for guess work during a consultation. The stylist must be very honest and sincere with the client, without insulting or belittling the person. Take time to ask the important questions and use the consultation as an opportunity to learn as much about the client's hair as possible. It is also a good time to explain what the natural hair care experience can offer the client. Adequate time for a braiding or locking consultation ranges from ten to thirty minutes. More time may be needed for clients with scalp disorders and hair loss. Clients with these special problems may want privacy. You should always offer the option of privacy to the client, particularly those with balding or scalp problems. Giving the client the option of privacy will remove any inhibitions that the client may have. Clients with scalp problems usually are very sensitive and feel vulnerable when displaying their hair problems. As a professional, your obligation is to help comfort, reassure, and encourage the client in order to build trust and confidence in your ability to provide the service. This is a key step in developing a bonding relationship between the stylist and client.

In a consultation setting, the stylist is focused on the client's perceived needs and personal expectations. A positive, unconditional reception of the client can build trust and confidence almost at the first meeting. According to "The Psychology of Hair and Cosmetology," unconditional positive regard communicates to clients acceptance without condition. This frees clients to be more expressive about their self-image and initiates an emotional, almost spiritual, bonding. Bonding with the client means developing a relationship, creating a connection personally and professionally during the first meeting. In the African tradition, this unconditional relationship is inherent in the braiding service.

Use the consultation as an opportunity to learn as much as possible about the client's chemical history, such as how many years of past chemical service, which products were used, and the frequency of service. In addition, a healthy discussion about the client's lifestyle, career, age and self-image can assist the stylist in determining the appropriate braided look or natural hairstyle. In choosing a braided look, the stylist must assist the client to define what is culturally aesthetic, as well as help decide what is professional and socially acceptable to them. Whatever style is chosen, the client should truly feel attractive and be effective professionally with the look.

A braided style should conform to the client's professional and social image. Sometimes during the interview the desired braid pattern may be in conflict with the client's profession or social image. The stylist can make suggestions that offer the client more diversity or simplicity. For example, a female police officer would have difficulty wearing a crown of **Goddess Braids** when in full uniform with a hat.

During the consultation, the stylist also takes into account the person's facial structure, height, and weight, before recommending a particular natural or braided style.

In choosing a braided look, the stylist must assist the client to define what is culturally aesthetic.

TYPES OF FACIAL STRUCTURES

As a natural hair care specialist, understanding facial types will enable you to create flattering styles which will enhance your client's best features. During the consultation, ask the client what she considers to be her best characteristics. Most people do not focus on the things they like about themselves; however, they can easily tell you what they consider to be flaws, imperfections, or negative facial characteristics.

As children, we have all experienced ridicule when an outstanding facial feature was highlighted and considered a negative characteristic. It does not matter whether it is the forehead, nose, ears, lips, or eyes that the client has internalized as being unattractive; what is important is that the stylist help the client choose braids or natural styles that flatter and affirm what they consider to be their positive features.

As a professional, it is your responsibility to assist the client in moving away from the emotional scars that have made him or her feel less than beautiful or acceptable.

It is important that the stylist help the client choose styles that flatter what they consider to be their positive features.

The following list is a general description of facial types that will assist you in choosing a flattering braid or natural hairstyle.

1. *Oval facial type—Traditional textbooks refer to this facial structure as the ideal facial type due to its evenly contoured or proportional features. The distance from the forehead to the chin is usually equally spaced. Generally, the forehead is slightly wider than the chin. This client can wear most braided or natural styles. Special considerations must be made for features such as wearing glasses, the nose size and shape, and the size and shape of lips.*

2. *Round facial type—This face is wide with a round or oval hairline. The chin is full and round. When styling, in order to create the illusion of thinness, add height when completing the finished look. Updo styles add length to the face. Asymmetrical styles that show the ears can create a slenderizing look for this facial type. Weaved or braided styles with waves or full curls help to create a balance and frame the face.*

3. *Square facial type—This face is wide with a square jaw line and an unusual or straight hairline. When styling, in order to create the illusion of length and to soften facial lines, full styles that frame the face around the forehead, temples, and jaw line are best. Wisps of hair or tapered fringe work best to soften any lines.*

4. *Diamond facial type—This face tends to be wide across the cheekbones. The forehead and chin are narrow. When styling, in order to minimize width across the cheekbones, create styles that are full around the forehead or jawline to help create an*

oval appearance. Full bangs or partial bangs will reduce the significance of a wide forehead. Keep the hair or braids close to the head along the cheekbones. Avoid updo styles and styles that move away from the cheeks or hairline.

5. *Heart-shaped facial type—This facial type consists of a wide forehead and a very narrow chin. The goal is to minimize the width of the forehead by styling the finished look with partial bangs or wisps of hair/braids that frame the face. This will add fullness around the chin.*

6. *Pear-shaped facial type—This facial type is recognized by its narrow forehead and wide chin or jaw. Soft fringes around the forehead will camouflage a small forehead without closing up the face. To give balance and fullness around the crown of the head, direct attention away from the narrow forehead. Styles that frame the cheekbones and are close or behind the ears can reduce a wide chin line.*

7. *Oblong facial type—This face is usually very long and narrow with small, hollow cheekbones. Creating full styles can make the face appear shorter or wider. The fullness must not be overpowering. Soft, partial bangs or wisps of curls along the face can soften facial lines. Hair/braids should not be very long—keep braid styles at a medium length. Avoid middle parts because they add length to a long, narrow face.*

> *Typical African features, should not have to be minimized or covered up. These are features that distinguish this ethnic group.*

Facial features that are specifically characteristic of African structure do not have to be minimized unless the client is uncomfortable or considers the feature a problem. Typical African features, such as high or large foreheads, wide/flat noses, big or full lips, and kinky textured hair, should not have to be minimized or covered up. These are features that distinguish this ethnic group. These features are traits that set this ethnic group apart from others, but they also make the people of this culture wonderfully unique. These features are attractive and acceptable within the African culture.

The entire purpose of redefining what is beautiful is to allow all people to define what they believe is beautiful and acceptable despite what they may have been conditioned to believe is "perfect." The braid stylist must be able to help the client "unlearn" these beliefs of perfection.

The following may assist the stylist when creating a finished look that will enhance unique features rather than simply camouflage them.

1. *Full or partial bangs, wisps, and fringes will minimize a large or wide forehead.*

2. *Center parts, updos, and styles that move away from the face can minimize a flat or wide nose because they tend to make the face look elongated.*

3. *By keeping braid styles close to the face, or by creating fullness around or behind the ears, protruding or large ears can be covered.*

Exhibit a professional and courteous attitude when speaking with a client in order to develop an open exchange.

THE CONSULTATION

The following steps are a guide to conducting a thorough consultation:

Step 1. Meeting the Client—Greet all new clients pleasantly. Smile and introduce yourself. Let the client know whether you are a locktician, barber, braider, receptionist, or owner/stylist. The client should be introduced to the actual braiding stylist and that designer should sit in on the consultation.

Exhibit a professional and courteous attitude when speaking with a client in order to develop an open exchange. Be honest and sincere without insulting the customer—even if the hair is abused, it is not your job to reprimand the person. Remember: clients come to you for your professional skills. You must be clear and direct. Maintain direct eye contact which conveys interest and sincerity. Looking at a person while he/she is talking shows that you are an "active listener" and that you are dedicated to fulfilling their needs.

Step 2. Seating the Client—The client should be offered a seat before the consultation begins. He/she should be seated comfortably in front of a mirror. It is also appropriate at this time to physically examine the hair and scalp. Stand next to or beyond the seated client while facing a mirror. In this position, you can maintain eye contact through the

TENDRILS
CLIENT PROFILE CARD

DATE

NAME

ADDRESS

CITY, STATE, ZIP

PHONE   WORK

OCCUPATION

BIRTHDATE   MONTH   DAY

SALON RECOMMENDATION BY

DO YOU TAKE ANY MEDICATION?

HAVE YOU EVER HAD YOUR HAIR BRAIDED? (YES OR NO)

CURRENT PRODUCTS USED

SHAMPOO   HOW OFTEN

COLOR   HOW OFTEN

PERM   HOW OFTEN

OTHER

HOME STYLING METHODS

BLOWER   DRY NATURALLY ☐

ROLLERS ☐   TYPE USED

OTHER   CURLING IRON

WHAT IF ANY PROBLEMS DO YOU HAVE WITH YOUR HAIR OR SCALP?

HAVE YOU EVER HAD ANY PROBLEMS WITH THE HAIR USED FOR EXTENSION—HUMAN OR SYNTHETIC?

DATE	SERVICE	PRICE

COMMENTS

Figure 4.1   Client profile card

mirror image while you consult. Through your body language, however, do not appear to stare or gaze for long periods of time. That may make the client feel intruded upon or uncomfortable.

Step 3. The Profile Card—A client profile card for the stylist's reference can be offered. This card should request basic information for background: the client's name, address, age, hair and chemical history, and home care products being used. Included in the information will be the client's hair care regime. Any special disorders or scalp problems should be noted. The client profile card will help the stylist to determine the condition of the hair. With the proper evaluation, the stylist can focus on correcting any styling problems that may occur. (Fig 4.1)

Step 4. Determine Client's Ideal Image—While the client is seated, show magazines or pictures of different braiding styles. This will start the dialogue about what the client is looking for in a hairstyle.

Step 5. Exchange of Dialogue—As previously mentioned, the consultation is a dialogue, not just a verbal communication to determine a desired result. It is an exchange of information that promotes success and satisfaction for both the client and stylist. The stylist must be an excellent listener by allowing the client time to talk. Repeat what the client has said or make a mental note. Do not interrupt. When a client says, "I really hate my hair," you say, "You really hate your hair. What do you hate about it?" Effective listening creates clarity and trust. Asking the right questions is very important.

Questions to ask during the interview:

- *What particular style do you have in mind?*
- *How do you see yourself with a braided style?*
- *What do you want from your hair?*
- *Describe your hair texture and length.*
- *What is your daily styling routine?*
- *What kind of work do you do?*
- *Will braiding your hair affect how others perceive you?*
- *Do you concern yourself with how others perceive you and your braided or natural hair?*

🌀 *What tools do you use to groom your hair?*

🌀 *What are your expectations from this braider or natural stylist?*

🌀 *What are the negative and positive experiences you have had with braids as a child or an adult?*

Step 6. Selecting Materials—When discussing a particular braiding design, the style may require that human hair or synthetic hair extensions be used. Various braiding styles require particular materials. The materials cost and pros and cons must be discussed in detail with the client.

Find out what past experiences, negative and positive, the client has had. Whatever problems the customer has had with a stylist in the past, remind the person that you will avoid similar mistakes. For example, if the client had problems with synthetic hair extensions, recommend styles that feature other extension materials, like human hair or yarn. Do not insist that the client try synthetic hair again just because you are doing the job. Avoid putting the client through the same experience—trial and error is too costly in this business.

Step 7. Hair Examination (Note: Protective gloves are optional)— The objective is to examine the texture of the potential client's hair. Take note of its density and length. By separating the hair at the scalp, look for the different wave patterns in the head. Pay close attention to areas where the hair is thinner, damaged, or broken. (These trouble spots should be noted on the profile card.) If the client suffers from a particular scalp disorder or is balding, make a notation and ask if the client is under any medical supervision or taking any medications.

Always remain sensitive to the client's discomfort when discussing such problems. Refer to Chapter 5 "How Hair Types and Structures Differ" for further discussion of hair characteristics.

Step 8. Scalp Abrasions—Examine the scalp for cuts or sores. Be careful not to irritate or scratch the affected area. Open sores should be avoided. If open sores are apparent, a dermatologist should be recommended. Again, remain sensitive to the care of the client.

Step 9. The Hairline—Brush a 1" hair section forward into the face to examine the hairline to see if it is receding or bald-

ing. If the hairline is damaged, certain braiding styles will be very difficult to execute. Avoid styles that place direct tension on the hairline or parting along the hairline.

Step 10. *Chemical History—Even though you are a natural hair care specialist, it is imperative that you learn what the client's experience has been with chemicals. Most clients looking for braided styles view braids as a means to repair hair damaged by chemicals. Braid styles can be stressful on the hair. If the hair has been weakened by past chemical treatments, the stylist must avoid certain styles until the client's hair is strong and healthy enough to withstand braided techniques. Chemical treatments have various effects on hair color, elasticity, and texture. The chemical history of the client will also have an impact on which natural shampoos and conditioners the stylist must use.*

It is imperative that you learn what the client's experience has been with chemicals.

If, after servicing your client, the client expresses concerns about the style, the tension, or the hairline, then it is obvious that you did not listen properly during the consultation. If the client is displeased in any way, you must take the responsibility for poor communications. On the other hand, if clients remain unclear during a consultation, trust your instincts and ask clients to defer to your judgement—after all, that is why the customer comes to you.

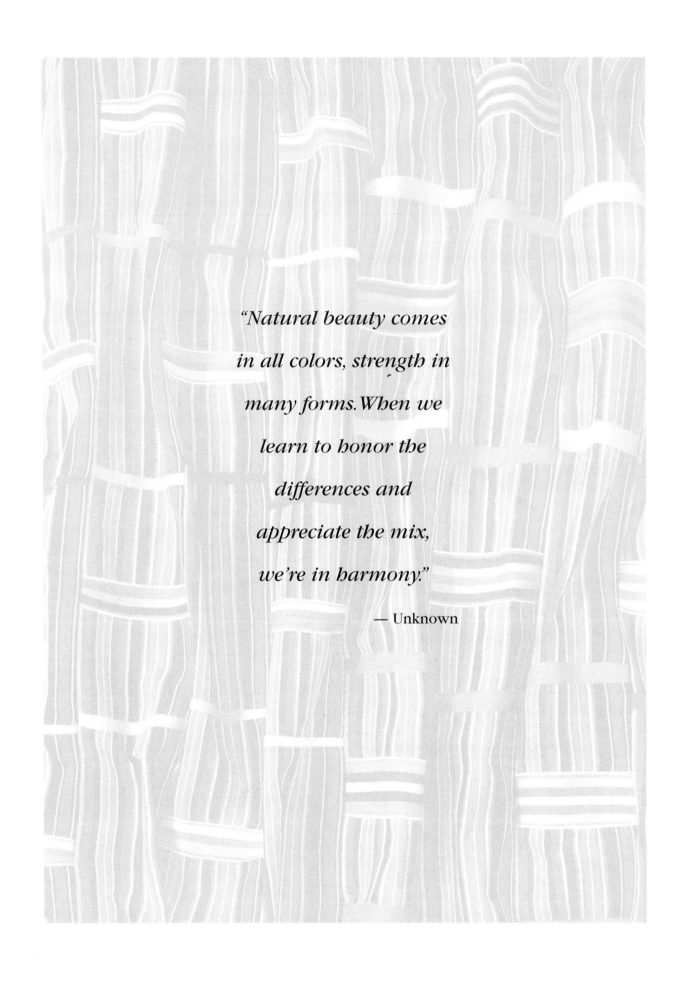

"Natural beauty comes in all colors, strength in many forms. When we learn to honor the differences and appreciate the mix, we're in harmony."

— Unknown

CHAPTER

5

How Hair Types and Structures Differ

KNOWLEDGE BOX

In this chapter you will learn:

1

Hair shapes

2

Structure of hair

3

Growth patterns

4

Composition of hair

5

Hair porosity and elasticity

INTRODUCTION

The primary function of hair is to insulate the body from the heat and the cold and to protect the head from injury and physical trauma. The secondary purpose of hair is for adornment. Having hair (or the lack of hair) may be pleasing to the eye.

But hair is considered an appendage of the skin. Hair is defined as a slender threadlike outgrowth of the epidermis of the skin and scalp. (Fig 5.1)

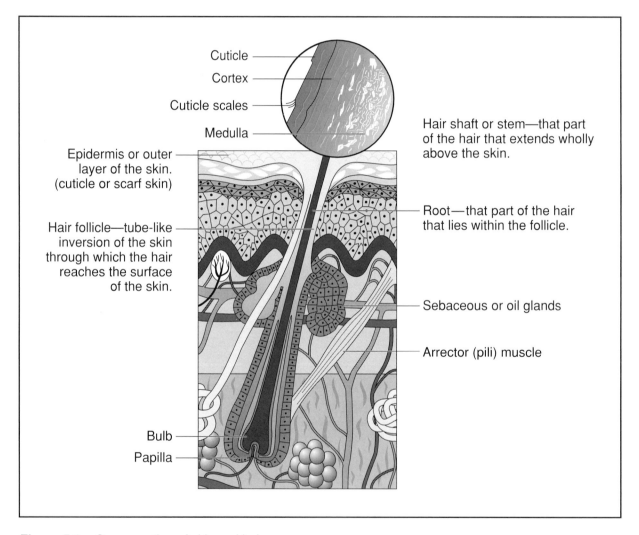

Cuticle

Cortex

Cuticle scales

Medulla

Hair shaft or stem—that part of the hair that extends wholly above the skin.

Epidermis or outer layer of the skin. (cuticle or scarf skin)

Hair follicle—tube-like inversion of the skin through which the hair reaches the surface of the skin.

Root—that part of the hair that lies within the follicle.

Sebaceous or oil glands

Arrector (pili) muscle

Bulb

Papilla

Figure 5.1   Cross-section of skin and hair

Hair is a cylinder of impacted protein, or keratinized cells, which are found in all horn growth such as nails and skin. (Fig 5.2)

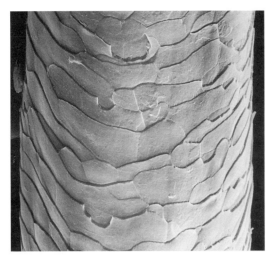

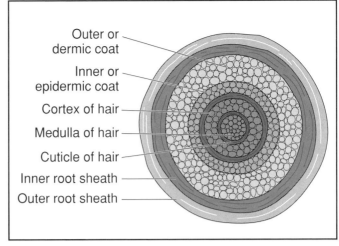

Outer or
dermic coat
Inner or
epidermic coat
Cortex of hair
Medulla of hair
Cuticle of hair
Inner root sheath
Outer root sheath

Figure 5.2 Magnified view of hair cuticle, which is composed of keratin.

Figure 5.3 Cross-section of the hair and follicle

DIVISIONS OF THE HAIR

Human hair is divided into two parts: the root and the shaft.

1. *Hair root—Hair structure beneath the skin surface; it lays within the follicle.*
2. *Hair shaft—Hair structure also known as the stem, that extends above the skin surface.*

Structure of Hair Root

The hair root is composed of three parts.

The hair root consists of the following:
1. follicle
2. bulb
3. papilla

Follicle

The **follicle** is the angular pocket-like depression in the scalp that encompasses the hair root. Every single strand of hair is enclosed in its own follicle. The follicle may vary in size, shape, and thickness depending on the genetic phenotype of the hair. The follicle directly determines texture and curl formation.

Other Hair Follicle Structures:

Arrector pili—An involuntary muscle under the hair follicle which allows the hair to contract and stand up when you are afraid or shivering cold. The skin looks like goose bumps.

Sebaceous glands—Little sac-like structures that provide the follicle with natural oils or **sebum**. Sebum adds luster and pliability to the hair and scalp. The production of sebum is directly associated with nutrition, emotional stress, and blood flow, as well as the impact of drugs and medication to the endocrine glands. Some studies show that most Africans produce more sebum than Caucasians and that the oils that reach the hair are derived from the scalp. However, because African type hair is tightly coiled, the natural oils are not distributed along the entire hair shaft. The result is dry, fragile hair.

Bulb

The **bulb** is a round structure at the very bottom of the hair root. The base of the root is hollowed out or concaved in order to fit over and cover the papilla.

Papilla

The **papilla** fits into the bulb at the base of the hair root. The hair papilla is filled with an ample supply of rich blood and nerve supply that nourishes the hair in order to stimulate growth and regeneration of the hair. It is through the papilla that the foods we eat provide nourishment to the hair bulb. A healthy papilla will generate hair cells in the bulb and produce new hair growth.

Structures Associated with Hair Follicles

The **arrector pili** is a small involuntary muscle attached to the underside of a hair follicle. Fear or cold causes it to contract and hair stands up straight, giving the skin the appearance of "goosebumps." Eyelash and eyebrow hair do not have arrector pili muscles.

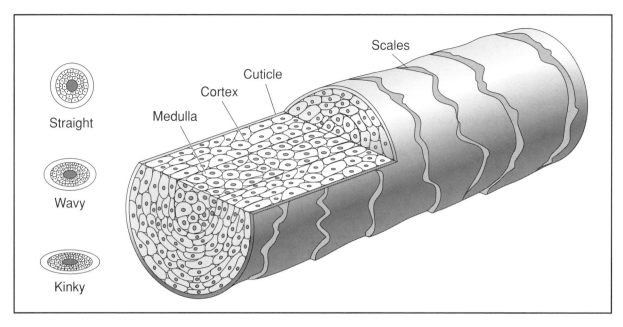

Figure 5.4 The hair shaft

Sebaceous, or oil, glands consist of little sac-like structures in the dermis. Their ducts are connected to hair follicles. Sebaceous glands frequently become troublemakers by overproducing and bringing on a common form of oily dandruff. Normal secretion of an oily substance from these glands, called sebum, gives luster and pliability to the hair and keeps the skin surface soft and supple. The production of sebum is influenced by diet, blood circulation, emotional disturbances, stimulation of endocrine glands, and drugs.

Endrocrine glands. The secretions of the endocrine glands influence the health of the body. Any disturbance of these glands can affect the health of the body and, ultimately, the health of the hair.

Drugs, such as hormones, can adversely affect the hair's ability to receive permanent waving and other chemical services.

Hair Shaft Structure

The hair shaft consists of three parts:

1. cuticle

2. cortex

3. medulla

The **cuticle** on the shaft is made up of dead protein called **keratin**, as well as amino acids such as cystine. It is the outer-most layer of the shaft that protects and seals the hair. The cuticle consists of flattened cells arranged like shingles on a roof. The scale-like cells overlap and lay close to the stem. When the cuticle is intact the hair stays healthy. When the cuticle is damaged through chemical processing, brushing, or heat, the edges of the cuticle begin to lift and separate from the shaft. Though the cuticle has seven to ten layers, once the cuticle lifts, it chips away from the shaft, the cortex and medulla are then exposed, which leads to breakage.

The **cortex** is the thickest part of the shaft. Long protein filaments, called **microfibrils**, are found in the cortex. Microfibrils make up the length of the hair. These fibers determine the strength, resilience, and moisture content of the hair. Disulfide and hydrogen bonds are small components that determine natural shape and form. Color is also determined in this middle layer. The disulfide bonds are strong and always want to return to their natural shape. The hydrogen bonds are weak and change easily when hair is shampooed or wet. The disulfide bonds can be broken down by permanents and chemical relaxers and are reformed with a new modified shape (straight or wavy) by neutralizing or stopping the reforming process. The hydrogen bond loses its shape when wet and reforms when heat is applied to the hair to dry. That is why hair is so fragile when wet—because the hydrogen bonds can be easily manipulated or broken.

Structurally, all hair is composed of the same elements.

The **medulla** contains components for color, moisture, elasticity, texture, and resilience. It is the inner-most core of the shaft. The melanin granules here determine the color of the hair. The medulla is porous, sponge-like, and contains protein, cystine and other amino acids, water, and fats. This core must be kept intact along with the cortex to have healthy hair.

VARIATIONS IN HAIR

Structurally, all hair is composed of the same elements. There are a few biochemical differences to explain the differences among different racial groups.

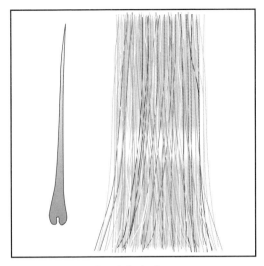

Figure 5.5a   Straight hair

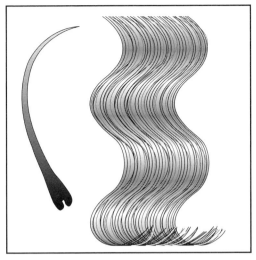

Figure 5.5b   Wavy hair

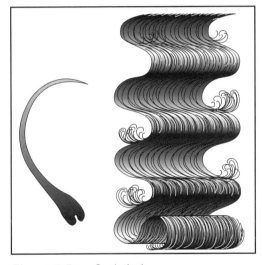

Figure 5.5c   Curly hair

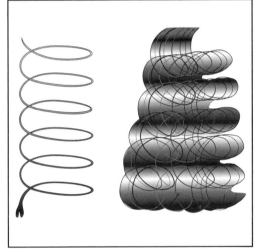

Figure 5.5d   Coily hair

In structure and form, hair is classified into three general configurations. As the hair grows away from the scalp, it assumes the shape and size of the hair follicle.

> *A cross section view of the hair under a microscope reveals that:*
> *1. straight hair is usually round*
> *2. wavy hair is oval to round*
> *3. curly hair is almost flat*
> *4. coiled or kinky hair is flat and spiraled*

Anyone can have straight, wavy, or curly hair, regardless of their race.

Structural Variation of Textured Hair

The phenotypic variations of hair based on racial groups is obvious. European hair generally looks wavy to straight. Asian hair appears to be generally straight. African hair is generally coiled. These very general classifications of texture are developed through genetic instructions. These genetic instructions create the amount of melanin in African skin, which gives skin its texture and color, as well as protects it from harmful ultraviolet (UV) rays. Genetically, the hair is programmed; the hair follicle is what determines the size and curl configuration or texture of the hair.

HAIR GROWTH CYCLES

The portion of the hair that is totally alive— the papilla, bulb, root, and follicle—is under the scalp.

Is hair alive? The answer is both yes and no. The hair that extends beyond the scalp and covers our head has no blood or nerve endings and therefore feels no pain when cut. But metaphysically and holistically, all hair is still connected to the body and therefore is a basic part of the life force. Hair responds to all of life's elements: the sun, water, wind, and temperature. Hair also reacts to the internal elements of the body: stress, emotional and physical shock, diet, drugs, and chemicals. The portion that we do not see is very much alive; hair has a spirit and life force that connects us with the universe. In the African tradition, some tribes believe that the hair is a spiritual transmitter. The portion of the hair that is totally alive— the papilla, bulb, root, and follicle—is under the scalp.

"The hair grows in cycles. It is a discontinuous process that varies based on race, heredity, sex, and age," says Debra Hare-Bey, owner of Red Creative Salon of NY, assistant editor of *Braids and Beauty* magazine and a master braider, in telephone conversation with the author. "I love to see textured hair grow. Whether it is a slow period or not, the cycle will continue if all the variables stay consistent. For example, nutrition. Drugs rob the body of its nutrients. The use of drugs or any stimulant will affect the nervous system and deteriorate the hair."

Three Cycles of Hair Growth

There are three distinct cycles to normal hair growth:

1. *Anagen growth*—*The period of development when the bulb is moving up through the follicle. The embryonic hair is being fed and nurtured at the root. The hair cell multiplies and expands, creating a new hair strand. This occurs between six months and six years.*

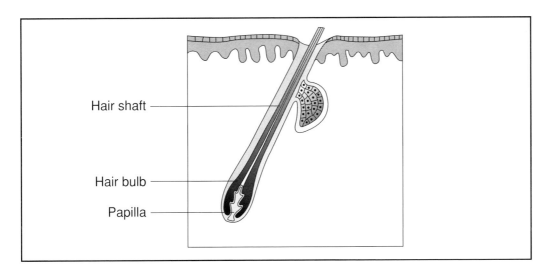

Figure 5.6a   Growth cycle of hair shaft

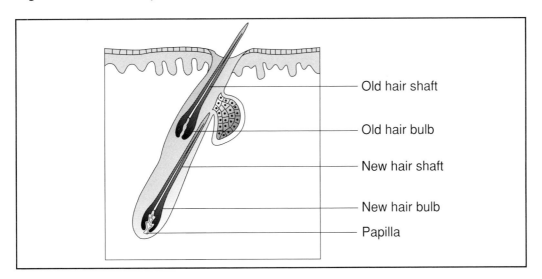

Figure 5.6b   Growth cycle of hair shaft

2. ***Catogen growth***—*The transition or resting stage. After two to six years of growing, the hair cells stop reproducing. The hair begins to lose moisture and separates from the papilla. This happens while a new hair begins to grow at the root.*

3. ***Telogen growth***—*The shedding stage. The old hair is pushed up to the scalp surface. The bulb is totally separate from the root. New hair cells divide and multiply, creating a new shaft. New hair sprouts to the surface of the scalp, pushing out old strands. This stage lasts a few weeks.*

The beauty of this entire process is that each hair strand is at a different stage at a particular time. At any given time, a strand is either growing, resting, or shedding. All the hair we see in the brush or comb is usually the hair that has naturally shedded. Fifty to 100 hairs per day can be in the shedding stage. (Fig 5.6 a, b)

**N
O
T
E**

— *Coily or spiral textured hair grows in a similar pattern; however, because it has a corkscrew pattern, it appears to grow slower. The flattened shaft gets thinner at every turn of the coil's bend. As the shaft bends, the flattened strand becomes weaker and more fragile. It is at this point, when stress through combing or brushing takes place, that the shaft breaks.*

HAIR QUALITY

When analyzing the condition of the hair, the stylist must be aware of the texture, porosity, and elasticity.

    ✂ ***Texture*** *refers to three qualities:*

        1. Curl configuration or shape—whether the hair is straight, wavy, curly, or coily.

C
A
U
T
I
O
N

— *Extremely porous hair stretches more than hair with poor porosity, such as overprocessed hair or hair damaged by chemical or color services—it tends to stretch like a rubber band and then break.*

2. *Diameter of the hair—refers to the size of the individual strands and the degree of coarseness, thickness, fineness, or thinness.*

3. *Feel of the hair—whether the hair feels greasy, hard, soft, smooth, coarse, or wiry.*

Porosity *refers to the hair's ability to absorb moisture or chemicals. Good porosity occurs when the hair shaft is lifted and can absorb normal amounts of moisture. Poor porosity occurs when the hair is resistant and absorbs the least amount of moisture. The cuticle layers lay flat and tight so that very little moisture is allowed into the shaft. The diameter of the strand (coarse, medium, or fine) will also determine the porosity. Coarse hair is often resistant; fine hair may often be extremely porous, absorbing moisture very easily.*

Elasticity *refers to the hair's ability to stretch and return to its original size and shape without breaking. Normal elasticity is springy and lustrous in appearance. Dry hair can stretch about 1/5 its length. Wet hair can stretch up to 50% of its length. When combing wet, coily hair, the hair can stretch up to twice its unencumbered length. Blow drying will also elongate the coil. Avoid extreme heat. The use of a hood dryer on loose twists can elongate the hair. The elasticity is often surprising to the client.*

HAIR TYPES

Textured Hair's Structural Differences

With the African hair type the follicle is spiral in shape. The hair shaft conforms to the shape of the follicle. It is the follicle that determines the configuration of coil. This is consistent throughout all major racial groups. The physical attributes of the shape and the amount of curl or coil is thought to be related to the cross-links in the cortex, which is genetically programmed during the molding of the hair shaft.

The textural difference in the frontal and crown regions have the greatest variety of diverse textures.

There are different degrees of coil, waves, and curls. The coil can be small, medium, or large in its spiral configuration. A small coil, for example, is tight in its winding pattern and may vary in other physical characteristics (such as fine or coarse to touch). The smaller the coil pattern, the greater the possibility of tangling (meshing for locks) and breakage when poorly groomed.

A medium coil or curl can also vary in its corkscrew pattern. Easier to groom, it tends to break less when combed. The meshing/locking process is slightly longer.

The longer coil or curl still requires proper grooming. Tangling or meshing still occurs and may take longer in the locking process.

The degrees and patterns of coils are almost endless. These are just general descriptions of textured hair. The professional locktician is the technician that addresses the specific needs of those clients that are interested in locking. They are experts on the subject of texture and the variety of techniques necessary for the varying hair textures to lock. Cultivating locks is truly a "hands on" art form. Cultivated locks are natural or chemically free hair, groomed in a systemized procedure to be symmetrical, circular, or manicured into a style. It is through the cultivation of locks that we can gather more information about the varying coil and curl patterns.

Coil patterns can differ on the same head. One client may display three or more textures throughout her head.

Generally, the texture of hair along the **occipital region** is tighter in its coil configuration; in some cases it may be dryer, more brittle and easier to break. The hair in this area tends to lock first during the locking process (refer to Chapter 10 "Braiding and Sculting Techniques"). There is a noted difference in texture along the **temporal** or sides of the head around the ear. This area may display a "softer" or fine coil. The hair is less brittle and the spiral pattern may vary from very tight or loose to a medium to large corkscrew pattern. The hair in this area generally locks next in the process. The textural difference in the frontal and crown regions have the greatest variety of diverse textures, ranging from fine, wiry waves to coarse, curly clusters or medium, grainy coils. The texture at the top of the head is often the last to lock. Neteb Ali, professional locktician and six-year owner of Trade Beads Lock Grooming in New York says, "Although we can only generalize about the varying textures, my experience with cultivating locks has shown that hair in varying parts of the head locks at different times because of the different degrees of coil. The hair at the crown may take longer to lock because heat is released from the top of the head. The heat may soften or relax the coil."

During the braiding service, the frontal area must be noted for its different or varying textures. Applying too much extension fiber can lead to breakage and permanent hair loss (refer to Chapter 6 "Scalp Diseases and Disorders").

The texture at the top of the head is often the last to lock.

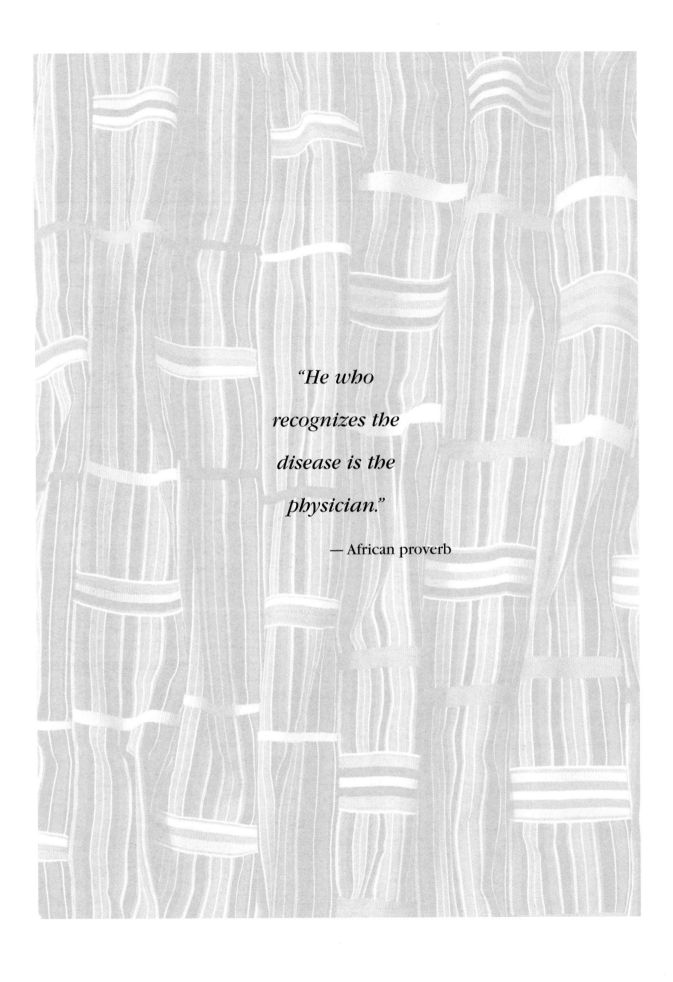

"He who

recognizes the

disease is the

physician."

— African proverb

CHAPTER

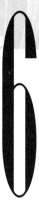

Hair and Scalp Diseases and Disorders

KNOWLEDGE BOX

In this chapter you will learn:

1

How to detect and treat dandruff

2

About chemical scalp and hair damage

3

About various types of alopecia

4

How to detect and treat seborrheic dermatitis

5

How to detect and treat keloidalis

6

About parasite and animal infections

INTRODUCTION

Hair loss can be traumatic emotionally and physically for men and women. A healthy and bountiful head of hair is directly correlated to one's self-esteem and general well-being. When hair loss occurs, the client's self-image is usually impaired.

> *It is important that the natural hair care specialist understands the nature of different types of hair loss for several reasons:*
> 1. *to help diagnose the problem*
> 2. *to service the client with the most effective treatment or camouflage*
> 3. *to refer the client to a medical professional if necessary*

Many clients that have a chemical history wrestle with hair breakage and scalp damage.

Hair care specialists should keep a list of dermatologists on hand that are experienced in treating African hair textures and their particular hair and skin disorders.

It is also necessary for the hair specialist to educate the client on proper grooming and styling techniques in order to help diminish the problem. If the affected area of hair loss is a recent problem for the client (occurred in the last three to six months), it may be possible for the hair care specialist to determine that the hair loss is the result of overprocessing, perms, or relaxers. Many clients that have a chemical history wrestle with hair breakage and scalp damage. Standard chemical treatments are harsh on the sponge-like scalp. The skin absorbs the chemicals and can react to it.

Also, when a client's hair begins to thin, break, or fall out, or when male-pattern baldness becomes apparent, the body is sending a signal that something is wrong. Hair loss can result from the following:

- *hereditary, male-patterned baldness due to inherited genes*
- *aging*
- *emotional stress*

- *sudden weight loss*
- *poor nutrition*
- *hormonal changes (pregnancy, menopause)*
- *surgery*
- *medications/drugs*
- *endocrine disorder, thyroid problems*
- *viral diseases, cancers, lupus*
- *infection due to improper sterilization*
- *excessive heat and chemical hair treatments*

The internal factors that may cause hair loss usually require professional medical attention for proper diagnosis. In some cases, a dermatologist will recommend a prescription shampoo and scalp treatment, which a client may request that you use instead of salon products. As with all products, read the labels and instructions before using on the client.

Hair loss that is directly related to hormonal imbalances, medications, vitamin deficiency, cancer, or HIV, can sometimes reverse itself with proper nutrition and expert care from a physician. If the medical condition can be arrested, many times the hair will return when the body heals. Clients that are living with cancer, lupus, HIV, diabetes and many other long-term, degenerative diseases are very sensitive—both physically and emotionally. The natural hair care specialist must be emotionally supportive and patient and must listen to clients' special styling needs. Often, natural braided styles must be created to camouflage, as well as diminish, the hair loss problem.

The natural hair care specialist must be emotionally supportive and patient and must listen to clients' special styling needs.

With hair loss, heavy thick braid extensions or extreme tension from cornrows or weaves must be avoided. These techniques will only accelerate the problem because the weight of extensions will weaken already fragile hair strands. Placing large amounts of hair extension on small amounts of thin, damaged hair can only cause further damage; it can be painful and will eventually lead to traction alopecia (discussed later in this chapter). In most cases, do not offer larger braid extension services (such as Casamas or corkscrews) during a hair growth transition period. This will avoid stress on damaged hair or scalp while new sparse hairs are returning. Using the "feed-in" method of cornrowing would best suit and protect hair in this transitional period.

For better results, offer non-extension braid services with nurturing hair and scalp treatments, scalp massages, and a supportive, positive outlook. Your attitude and disposition will help the client relax and eventually build trust in your ability to nurture and groom his or her hair. Another alternative for major hair loss would be to offer the client a stylish, contemporary wig. This will allow you to continue hair treatments without causing styling stress on affected areas of the scalp. Styling and cutting a wig is a regular service you may offer clients with special needs.

Offer all of the possibilities to your client including the natural or braided styles that will encourage hair growth.

Hair growth does not occur overnight. Inform your client that whatever caused the hair loss problem took months or years to manifest. It will take much more to stop the problem and for the client's hair to return. If the scalp is badly scarred or chemically burned, or if the hair papilla (near bulb of hair strand) is totally destroyed, permanent hair loss will occur. Never create false hope. Be realistic with clients. Offer all of the possibilities to your client including the natural or braided styles that will encourage hair growth and enhance the client's appearance.

DISORDERS OF THE HAIR

Canities is the technical term for gray hair. Its immediate cause is the loss of natural pigment in the hair. There are two types:

1. *Congenital canities exists at or before birth. It occurs in albinos and occasionally in persons with normal hair. A patchy type of congenital canities may develop either slowly or rapidly, depending on the cause of the condition.*

2. *Acquired canities may be due to old age, or onset may occur prematurely in early adult life. Causes of acquired canities may be worry, anxiety, nervous strain, prolonged illness, or heredity.*

Ringed hair is alternate bands of gray and dark hair.

Hypertrichosis, or hirsuties, means superfluous hair, an abnormal development of hair on areas of the body normally bearing only downy hair.

Treatment is to tweeze or remove by depilatories, electrolysis, shaving, or epilation.

Trichoptilosis is the technical term for split hair ends. Treatment is that the hair should be well oiled to soften and lubricate the dry ends. The ends may also be removed by cutting.

Trichorrhexis nodosa, or knotted hair, is a dry, brittle condition including formation of nodular swellings along the hair shaft. The hair breaks easily and there is a brushlike spreading out of the fibers of the broken-off hair along the hair shaft. Softening the hair with conditioners may prove beneficial.

Monilethrix is the technical term for beaded hair. The hair breaks between the beads or nodes. Scalp and hair treatments may improve the hair condition.

Fragilitas crinium is the technical term for brittle hair or split ends. The hairs may split at any part of their length. Conditioning hair treatments may be recommended.

CHEMICAL DAMAGE

As a naturalist you will not, by law, be allowed to apply chemical altering services. However, it is your responsibility to understand how they work on textured hair.

The factors that cause hair loss usually stem from improper chemical relaxing and perm applications.

The external factors that can traumatize the scalp and cause hair loss usually stem from improper chemical relaxing and perm applications. Most African-American women have straightened their textured hair with chemical relaxers—it is the most popular form of styling. About 90% of African-American women relax their hair at one time or another. There are two basic types of chemical straighteners. One is sodium hydroxide or lye perm; the other is guanidine hydroxide and lithium hydroxide relaxers or "no lye" perms. Due to the instability of the guanidine hydroxide relaxers, an "activator" or calcium hydroxide is added to the base to protect new growth of textured hair. "No lye" perms, as they are called commercially, dominate the retail market. They are the most popular because they claim to be mild, safe, gentle relaxers. These claims are misleading.

The sodium hydroxide relaxers (lye perms) have a high *pH* (potential hydrogen—the degree of acid mantle in the hair and scalp). The optimum neutral pH level for hair is 7. The lower the number on the pH scale the more *acidic* the content. A pH higher than 7 indicates the *alkaline* level. The highest level on the pH scale is 14. Sodium hydroxide relaxers are the most caustic and reactive because of the high pH levels, ranging about 12-14 on the pH scale, and are potentially dangerous to the hair and scalp. When this type of relaxer touches the scalp, forehead, ear or neck, burning irritation may occur. Before applying this type of relaxer, a pre-application of *petrolatum* is required to protect the skin and scalp.

The lower the number on the pH scale the more acidic the content.

These highly alkaline relaxers or *base relaxers* require that the stylist use an emollient such as petrolatum, because manufacturers anticipate chemical burns to the skin. The other type of relaxer referred to as **no base relaxers**, may be composed of guanidine hydroxide (no lye). They are marketed as having no need to use a protective petrolatum base. However, in some cases some burning may occur with a no base, no lye relaxer, although chemical burning is less frequent.

If these products are used, they should be applied carefully and with caution. Despite their claims, superficial chemical burns are very common, especially with the alkali relaxers. Irritation, blistering, scabbing, and permanent hair loss does happen, especially if chemical burns are experienced repeatedly over a long period of time, destroying the hair follicle.

The most frequently noted side effect from using chemical relaxers is hair breakage. Anyone who has had a relaxer applied to their hair has experienced some type of breakage. Hair breakage is most common at the **suboccipital** nape of the neck, where the chemical is often first applied and is exposed to the hair for the longest time. The frontal and temporal hair lines are secondary locations of damage because of long exposure to the chemical and overlapping process during touch-up services.

For most women, touch-up service is much too frequent for chemically treated hair—usually occurring every three to four weeks. This is not enough time to allow new growth of natural hair. Noted dermatologist Dr. Wesley Wilborn of Atlanta, GA, believes that frequent re-touches are harmful.

He says, "The relaxer invariably will overlap onto previously treated hair, causing resultant, irreparable damage to the hair shaft and subsequent breakage."[1]

A dipilatory effect may occur from the improper use of a chemical relaxer, says Dr. Wilborn. The hair literally "melts away" when the cosmetologist incorrectly chooses the wrong relaxer or leaves the product on too long. What the cosmetologist must be aware of is that all chemicals cause some kind of side effect, and that it is their responsibility to minimize the occurrence when using these products.

Factors that affect the degree of breakage from relaxers:

- *strength of relaxer*
- *application time*
- *effective removal (neutralizing shampoo)*
- *hair texture, phenotype*
- *desired finished look*

Many of the no base relaxers are marketed for home use. Consumers buy the home kit in order to apply the relaxer themselves. Inevitably, the consumer will overlap or overprocess the hair. Most people will overlap in the sections of the head that cannot be easily reached, such as the nape and crown. Although no base relaxers are milder to the scalp, when used improperly the chemicals can create breakage and scalp damage.

So called "kiddie perms" are another popular chemical service offered as a home kit. Beautiful young girls with shiny bone straight hair are displayed on the boxes. The advertising is aimed toward vulnerable youths who want to look like the girls on the box. But what the advertising is really saying to young children is that you are more acceptable with straight hair.

In the 1970s and 1980s, "Jheri curls" and "California Curls" or thioglycolate perms were extremely popular. These chemical services offered African-American men and women other styling options. First, the natural texture had to be removed or chemically straightened. Then the hair was rolled and saturated with an oxidizing agent or neutralizer to reshape the wave patterns, creating a loose curl. This two-step procedure lost its populari-

Although no base relaxers are milder to the scalp, when used improperly the chemicals can create breakage and scalp damage.

---

[1] Wilborn, Dr. Wesley, <u>Disorders of Hair Growth in African-Americans,</u> 1994, 395.

**C
A
U
T
I
O
N**

Five- to ten-year-old girls should avoid all relaxers. The breakage and scalp damage can be irreversible on such young skin. Parents may mean well, but in most cases they are not professionals, nor skilled to use such caustic chemicals. Hair loss at a tender age can shatter a child's self-image.

**N
O
T
E
S**

You can educate the client to understand the seriousness of chemical relaxers. As a professional, you can make the difference in a client's self-discovery and the self-image of young girls, especially. You should aim to work with *texture not* against *it. Soften textured hair instead of totally removing it. That is the best approach. Do not aim to break the wave pattern.*

ty because of the severe scalp damage and breakage that it caused. The active ingredient, ammonium thioglycolate, was strong and depleted moisture from the hair. To maintain the curled style, the client was required to replace moisture frequently with emollients that sealed in moisture and kept the hair wet and tacky (sticky). Often people would cover their heads with plastic bags and shower caps to retain the moisture. Hair breakage occurred during the straightening process, or if the hair was not kept hydrated. The same factors that affect breakage for relaxers hold true for curl or wave systems, only straighteners are stronger when dry. Curled or wavy hair is stronger when moist.

Many clients reported that when they had a curly perm, their hair was healthier and grew more rapidly. One client actually said that the curl made her hair grow. But it was not the chemical service that appeared to promote hair growth, it was the moisturizing gels, sprays, and lotions that kept the hair wet and moist that aided in protecting the hair. Although the popularity of the curl perms has declined, use of moisturizing agents have not.

Braid and lock moisturizers are readily available because they contain what textured hair needs to stay healthy—oil and moisture. Naturally textured hair that is kept moist will comb out more easily, prevent breakage from combing and brushing, and will grow longer.

N
O
T
E
S

Refer to Chapter 8 "Shampoos, Conditioners, Herbal Treatments, and Rinses" for a list of oils to use for various treatments. The following oils have little or no side effects on clients that experience seborrhea: petrolatum, mineral oil (synthetics have no therapeutic value), lecithin vegetable glycerine, propylene glycol (synthetic gylcerine), evening primrose oil, jojoba oil, and shea butter. Refer to the herbs and oils list for further information on using these oils.

DANDRUFF

The outermost layer of the scalp, the epidermis, continually sheds and replaces dead skin cells. A natural shedding of these small skin cells is a normal human occurrence and should not be confused with dandruff. Normal shedding is a light powdery form of skin cells that disappear when the hair is washed or brushed. **Dandruff**, medically known as **pityriasis**, is characterized by large scales or flakes from the scalp.

Dandruff is usually accompanied by an itching sensation and a scattering of scales on the shoulder, hair, scalp, and sometimes eyebrows. This excessive shedding of the **epithelial cells** (surface layers) is visible and large in size because it is an accumulation of the buildup of the normal shedding process and of the large flaky scales. This creates a sluggish condition of the scalp and dandruff occurs.

> ### *There are two types of dandruff:*
>
> 1. ***Pityriasis capitis simplex**—The dry type associated with flaking, scattered scales, and itching. It is very visible on hair and shoulders.*
>
> 2. ***Pityriasis steatoides**—Greasy or waxy type. Large scales are combined with sebum causing the scales to stick to the scalp in white creamy patches. When the waxy, creamy scales are removed with a comb, bleeding or oozing sebum may result. Medical treatment is required.*

Dandruff is usually accompanied by an itching sensation and a scattering of scales.

Internal factors for dandruff caused by a sluggish scalp:

- *poor circulation or metabolism*
- *hormonal imbalance*
- *poor nutrition*
- *lack of water*
- *stress and tension*
- *glandular problems*
- *biochemical changes to the scalp*

External factors that induce dandruff or sluggish scalp:

- *lack of proper cleansing*
- *infrequent shampooing*
- *topical medication ointments*
- *oils or creams that irritate the scalp*
- *increased activity of bacteria or fungi*
- *poor scalp stimulation*
- *high pH in water*
- *high pH shampoos*

The nature of dandruff is still uncertain. A yeast-like organism has been found in the dandruff scales; however, studies have not been conclusive to its origin. Medical authorities do consider dandruff to be contagious. Cross-contamination can occur by the common use of brushes and combs, scarfs and hats, and any other shared articles for the head. Therefore, it is important that the natural hair care specialist take all the necessary sanitation precautions when servicing a client with this disorder. Sanitize all tools that come into contact with clients.

Dandruff Treatments

Commercial dandruff shampoos all claim to treat the problem of dandruff. These shampoos are usually made with tar solutions that temporarily address the problem. The flaking generally re-appears within two to three days, which would require frequent shampooing to control or minimize the problem. For African-American hair types, daily shampooing is very drying and stressful to their hair as well as impractical. Therefore, the stylist must look for products that offer longer, more effective results or that enhance commercial shampoos by adding natural extracts to aid the problem.

Shampoos, conditioners, hot oil treatments, or ointments that contain the following substances have been noted to be effective as anti-dandruff products:

1. *Selenium—Effective in a shampoo that contains sulfur, amino acids (cystine, cystini), herbs such as coltsfoot, horsetail, rosemary, sage; or vegetable oils such as evening primrose, jojoba, or peppermint (see herbal chart page 136).*

2. *Sulfur—Found in the keratin fibers of protein in the hair and scalp. A deficiency of sulfur can weaken or impair the mucous membranes of the sebaceous gland (sebum) which can lead to dandruff and seborrhea, or hair loss.*

3. *Horsetail, coltsfoot, nettle, rosemary, and sage—These botanicals are rich in sulfur and amino acids; vitamin B complex (panthenol and inositol) increase blood circulation and provide nutrients that can be absorbed into the scalp to diminish seborrhea (excessively oily scalp).*

4. *Garlic or garlic extracts—It has anti-inflammatory properties and is used for its anti-fungal and antiseptic properties. It has a strong odor.*

For African-American hair types, daily shampooing is very drying and stressful to their hair as well as impractical.

How to Service Dandruff Problem

A client with a dandruff problem may be treated by using the following procedure:

1. Drape client, covering clothing and hands.
2. Examine scalp; note where the concentration of buildup is.
3. Gently brush or comb scalp to stimulate blood flow and lift scales. Avoid applying pressure. If blood or sebum seepage occurs, stop. There may be seborrheic dermatitis.
4. Shampoo with medicated or special shampoo designed to minimize the condition on the scalp.
5. Allow shampoo to remain on the scalp. Five to twenty minutes is generally enough time. Rinse thoroughly.
6. The second shampoo should be a conditioning shampoo for the hair. Massage in shampoo with circular movements to soothe and stimulate. If the hair is braided, avoid disrupting the style. Use smaller circular movements that are slightly deeper in touch. Rinse thoroughly.
7. Apply warm herbal rinse or hot oil treatment or anti-dandruff lotions to parted small sections of the scalp. Deep conditioners can be applied to the hair.
8. Slowly massage into the scalp.
9. Place cotton around the head to protect eyes and clothing. Place plastic cap on the head.
10. A hair steamer or heating cap can be placed on the head. Apply heat for fifteen to twenty minutes.
11. Rinse thoroughly; towel dry hair.
12. Lightly spray hair or braid with a finishing rinse or comprehensive lotion or oil to coat hair for an easy comb-out.
13. Groom and style. Blow drying may be used at warm air temperature.

SEBORRHEIC DERMATITIS

This is an inflammatory reaction to some commonly used hair products. It is the abnormal increase of sebum secretion on the scalp. Seborrhea may be induced by the following:

- lanolin
- soy bean oil
- wheat germ oil
- lecithin
- castor oil
- squalene

By simply avoiding certain hair products containing these ingredients, the problem may reverse itself. Natural ingredients that help control seborrhea dermatitis for natural styles are:

- *pure jojoba oil*
- *rose hip seed oil*
- *glycerine*
- *almond oil*
- *lavender*

Seborrheic dermatitis looks like wet dandruff. It consists of white, creamy, yeast-like film or patches that coat the scalp. However, unlike dandruff, there is little flaking. The oil discharge of sebum and skin scales adhere to the scalp. Although the scalp may be oily, in African hair types the hair still may be dry. Therefore, daily shampooing is not recommended. Suggest that a client wash their hair once a week with a medicated or anti-dandruff shampoo. The shampoos should remain on the scalp for at least ten minutes, applied directly to the scalp. Avoid strong medicating cleansing products because they may not benefit the dry hair.

If the problem persists, a dermatologist may be recommended. Follow all prescribed medical instructions. Treatment procedures are the same as the dandruff procedures mentioned previously. In some cases, heavy oil, i.e., olive oil, can stimulate the problem. Avoid heavy oils when treating this dermatitis.

ALOPECIA

Alopecia (al-oh-pee-shee-ah) is the general term for a variety of abnormal hair loss conditions.

I have had personal experiences with this condition and for many years have experimented with commercial and natural treatments. With some success over a long period of time, including lifestyle changes, locking my hair, and changes in my diet, I have restored growth to very thin and small bald patches in my hair.

There are more than twenty different types of alopecia disorders. These excessive hair loss problems should not be confused with normal hair shedding. It is estimated that the average life cycle of a hair strand is four to five years. Yet, no one is quite certain of this number. A varying amount of hair will shed daily, creating a continuum for new hair growth. This shedding process is altered by a variety of factors:

- *gender*
- *age*
- *hair type*
- *nutrition (protein, iron, zinc or essential/fatty acid deficiencies)*
- *heredity*
- *physical health (hormonal changes, especially thyroid, postpartum shedding)*
- *emotional health (psychological stress or trauma)*
- *drugs or chemical ingestion*

However, the average daily hair loss is about 50 to 100 telogen strands of hair.

The scalp is filled with three types of hairs. Hair that is actively growing is anogen hair. Hair that has stopped growing but is strong is catagen hair. Hair that is in a resting or telogen phase stops growing and begins to **atrophy** or shrink and fall out excessively.

However, this process can be accelerated when external or internal trauma takes place. When the body or the spirit has been traumatized, alopecia of some form will occur, signaling to the stylists that special services should be rendered. Hair loss due to emotional stress will reverse itself naturally once the stress is alleviated. But alopecia due to hormonal imbalances or physical stress can be permanent.

Types of Alopecia

There are three distinct types of alopecia:

1. *Alopecia senilis (se-nil-is)—Loss of hair or balding that occurs with old age. It is permanent and is inherent to aging skin and poor blood circulation. Follicles atrophy with age.*

2. *Alopecia prematura (pre-mah-chor-ah)—Balding occurs at a slow pace with a thinning process usually during middle age (fifteen to thirty-five years old). This type of balding occurs when the hair falls out and is replaced by smaller, weaker hairs (**vellus** hairs) often found on the crown or front of the head.*

3. *Alopecia areata (air-ee-ah-tah)—Refers to the sudden or sometimes unrecognized falling out of hair in patches or spots. Bald spots can be round or irregular in shape and vary in size from 1/2" to 4" in diameter. The patches are usually lighter in color (often pale) because of the poor blood supply to the area.*

Alopecia due to hormonal imbalances or physical stress can be permanent.

Alopecia areata is usually triggered by trauma to the nervous system and circulatory system in the **lymphatic** system, which aids in nourishing and detoxing the blood cells, kidneys, glands, and large intestines. Diseases like scarlet fever, typhoid fever, syphilis, Hodgkin's disease, or anemia can trigger this kind of disorder.

Alopecia areata is caused by a variety of abnormal physical conditions which affect the scalp condition or health. External treatment to stimulate blood flow will help to repair the scalp. Slow therapeutic massage is recommended to increase blood flow and to create a nurturing environment, which helps the client to relax.

Massages with **aromatic oils** and herbs are helpful and create calmness through the **olfactory** systems (smell). **Aromatherapy** with essential oils has been recorded since the 12th Dynasty Egypt to heal and nurture the body. Stimulating oils are:

- *peppermint*
- *rose hip seed oil*
- *lavender*
- *eucalyptus*
- *rosemary*
- *thyme*
- *spearmint*
- *sandalwood*

Alopecia areata is caused by a variety of abnormal physical conditions which affect the scalp condition or health.

How to Treat Alopecia

Alopecia can be treated using the following eleven-step procedure:

1. *Preheat oil needed for the hair treatment.*
2. *Shampoo once to remove surface debris from hair or braid.*
3. *Apply warm oil to scalp in small amounts, section by section.*
4. *Massage the scalp, slowly and rythmically, kneading, stroking and rolling and squeezing gently. Avoid disturbing braid extensions or tangling hair. Focus on the scalp.*
5. *Once the oil is distributed evenly, place a cotton strip around the entire head to avoid dripping into the client's eyes.*
6. *Place a damp towel or plastic cap on the head to retain moisture.*
7. *Using a hair steamer or heating cap, apply heat for twenty minutes. A conditioning rinse may be applied to the hair.*
8. *Apply mild conditioning or medicated shampoo for the second cleansing.*

9. Rinse; towel dry.

10. Lightly spray hair or braids with a finishing rinse or comprehensive lotion to coat the hair for manageability.

11. Groom; blow dry with low, warm air for braided style.

Traction Alopecia

This is the most common balding disorder among young African-American women and girls. Many suffered with this problem in early adolescence. Traction baldness occurs when the hair is pulled too tightly. The hair is literally pulled out of the follicle, taking with it the hair root and the bulb. Destroying the hair shaft may cause white bumps and pus or scaling to occur around the affected area. If the tight pulling continues over a long period of time, permanent scarring or balding will develop.

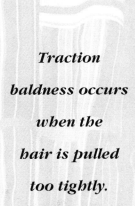

Traction baldness occurs when the hair is pulled too tightly.

It takes about one to three years for the bald spot to develop. But if the client continues to style or groom their hair the same way, day after day, without altering the tension, traction alopecia can begin very rapidly, sometimes within weeks. Hair loss is often apparent in the frontal and temporal regions of the head. Also the nape of the neck can be affected by traction alopecia, depending upon how the hair is styled and the hair texture.

Traction alopecia is directly related to improper grooming techniques and hairstyling practices. The main culprits to this disorder are tight braids, ponytails, and the worst offenders: sponge rollers. (Figs 6.1 and 6.2)

Braids and Traction Alopecia

Initially, all braids create a small amount of tension on the hair. However, when properly starting the braid style, cornrows, or extensions, there should not be pain, discomfort, or irritation to the scalp in any way. The braid stylist must always remember the basic concept of the service, which is to nurture and groom.

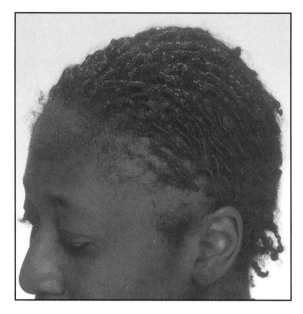

Figure 6.1 Close crop highlight—traction alopecia, temporal region

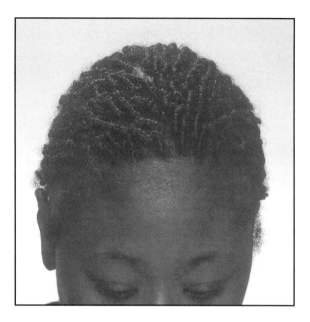

Figure 6.2 Close crop—traction alopecia, frontal region

🌀 *Improper tension—This occurs when starting the braid. Too often braiders start the braid very tightly to apply extension to the hairline (frontal and temporal regions), trying to gather the fine or broken strands of hair while keeping the extension taut.*

🌀 *Excessive amounts of hair extension—Applying too much extension material in disproportion to the number of strands in the sectioned hair can cause excessive tension on the natural hair. The extension material becomes too heavy for small amounts of natural hair, particularly when the hair begins to grow out from the base. When it grows away from the base, the large, heavy braid extension is hanging from three to four strands of natural hair, causing tension.*

🌀 *Wearing the braid too long—Three months is the average length of time for an extended braid style. If worn longer, breakage may occur. As the natural hair grows, the extension grows away from the base, then starts to pull and stress the scalp area. It also rubs and erodes the exposed area which can lead to balding and breakage.*

🌀 *Pulled back hair or braid styles—Braid styles that are constantly pulled back away from the face contribute to the tension. Single braids or cornrows that are always stressing the hairline need to be worn down occasionally to relieve the tension on the scalp. (Fig 6.3) Braid styles that are up all the time are also detrimental to the scalp. They should not be worn for more than two months. Try to style the braids so that they can be loosened nightly, or worn down to relieve the stress on the scalp.*

🌀 *Pustules—Pustules are small white pimples that seep pus. This is a direct result of tension from excessive pulling, causing lack of circulation. If scratched or irritated, the pustules may become infected. This condition may require medical attention.*

🌀 *Ponytails—Young girls and very busy working women find it easier to simply get a rubber band or some elastic and pull the hair back into a ponytail. It appears to be neat, quick and easy, but is also very damaging to the hair and scalp if it is too tight and worn constantly.*

It is the pulling tension from ponytails that affects the scalp. It is the very slick, sleek updos that are very popular and contribute to this problem. When putting in a ponytail or updo, give a little slack to the style. The braid stylist will know if the hair is too tight if the client's eyes and skin are pulled taut into an almond shape and are distorted to look more Asiatic. Some people jokingly refer to the ponytail as the Black woman's face lift.

Hair accessories associated with this style can be problematic too. Rubber bands, elastic clips, bows and clamps are all attractive and easy to use but can be damaging to the hair. When in doubt, avoid all rubber bands or elastic ties. Some elastic ties are covered in cotton and are more appropriate when not doubled around the braid. Also, remember to instruct the client to remove the ponytail at the end of the day. This will relieve the scalp of any tension.

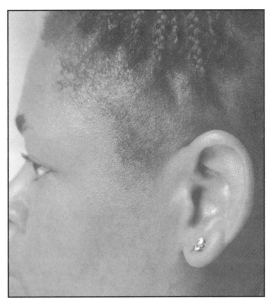

Figure 6.3 Traction alopecia with braid pulled up

One day I was getting breakfast at a nearby restaurant. Ahead of me was a lovely five or six-year-old girl and her mother. Both were dressed for the day and the little girl's hair was exceptionally well groomed. Her hair was neatly parted and sectioned into six or seven plaits, each neatly tied with elastic white bows. As I admired her hair, I noticed the skin folded at the crown (top) of her head. The elastic bows were pulled so tight that the skin actually creased, making a fold in the skin! I was so alarmed that I turned to the mother and told her that the bands were extremely tight and pointed out the affected area. Needless to say, the mother was not very pleased, but friendly enough to immediately loosen one of the bands. That was an uncomfortable moment for the child, but she was so relieved when it was loosened—and so was I.

🌀 *Sponge rollers—Sponge rollers are the worst hair setting product on the market (in the author's opinion and after years of witnessing the damage they have caused clients). They have destroyed millions of women's hairlines forever. The most common affected area is the frontal and temporal regions; however, depending on the style and hair texture, the occipital area or nape can be badly damaged as well.*

This is a situation where women sacrifice healthy, bountiful hair for the sake of fashion. These women totally ignore the warning signs of hair loss and thinning, continue to practice improper grooming, and wearing damaging hairstyles. Pam Ferrell, author of Where Beauty Touches Me, *noted on one of her many trips to West Africa, that it was very common to see young girls and women with hairlines as far back as two inches. She attributes this to abusive practices that are taught from one generation to another.[2] The same holds true for styling or curling the hair with sponge rollers. Our peers and mothers used them, so many continue to use them.*

The real problem with these rollers is that there is no "give" when winding the hair around the pink sponge. These rollers will create an excellent tight curl, but also create tension and stress on affected areas. Once the hair is unwrapped, hair is always found stuck on the sponge, even with end paper used to protect the hair strands. Sponge rollers are soft and therefore it appears that it is easier to sleep when they are used, but while sleeping the sponge is rubbing and eroding the hairline. If one does not pay close attention, a bald spot will begin to appear. If ignored, the hair loss can be permanent.

Women ignore the warning signs of hair loss by continuing to wear damaging hairstyles.

---

[2] Ferrell, Pam, <u>Where Beauty Touches Me</u>, Washington, DC: Cornrows & Co. Publication, 1993, 40.

When you have a client with traction alopecia, which is a clear sign of hair abuse, it is the stylist's responsibility to re-educate the client. Hopefully, they will teach their daughters how to properly groom and manage their hair in order to stop the abuse.

Steps to Take with Traction Alopecia

There are five steps you should take when dealing with clients' alopecia:

1. *Learn the client's history and styling practices and note them on the client's profile card during the consultation.*
2. *Point out all the areas that are affected and note them.*
3. *Try to determine whether the damage appears to be permanent and insist that the client stop any abusive behavior to the hair.*
4. *Suggest camouflage styling techniques to help the client feel and look better.*
5. *Once tension is removed and nurturing treatments are applied, new hair may come back. However, it will be intermittent growth.*

When you have a client with traction alopecia, it is the stylist's responsibility to re-educate the client.

FOLLICULITIS KELOIDALIS

This scalp disorder is common among young African-American men. It is also known as Acne Keloidalis or Perifolliculitis Keloidalis Occipital (PFKO) and commonly referred to as "razor bumps." This disorder is the chronic inflammation, irritation, and infection of the hair follicle. This infection leads to scarring or lesions, usually found in the occipital region of the head or the back of the neck. The scarring usually occurs in areas where a razor or an electric liner is used to enhance the hairline.

In the early stage of this scalp disorder soft papules (pimples) rise, harden with time and eventually form keloidal tissue. The skin has been traumatized by the repeated use of the unsanitized razor or liner, therefore creating an infection of the follicle.

Currently with the close cuts like "fades," "caesars," and "bald cuts," where razors and liners repeatedly touch the skin to remove coiled, curly hair, this disorder has increased in its occurrence. More women are experiencing this disorder because of the increasing popularity of short new cuts.

> ### Two heredity factors contribute to this severe keloidal scarring:
>
> 1. Coiled/curly hair—The tight kink or coil formation of the follicle determines the hair shape. Consequently, the curl shaft, when cut close, pierces and re-enters the skin, forming pimples or papules.
> 2. Large numbers of African-Americans are genetically prone to keloids. When the skin tries to heal itself after the razor cut, instead of creating a scab, the skin cells produce inflamed tissues. The soft papules dry and harden, leaving raised skin tissue or keloid.

Those prone to scarring should avoid fades or bald cuts and allow the hair to grow a little fuller and away from the scalp.

This problem can be avoided by the client not having their hair cut close or their necks lined. Those prone to scarring should avoid fades or bald cuts. The client should always allow the hair to grow a little fuller and away from the scalp. Wearing hair twisted or in locked styles are great alternatives.

A dermatologist must be recommended if the infection is active. A typical and/or systemic antibiotic is usually required to aid the healing process.

Remember to always sanitize tools before every service. Infection of the follicle can be avoided if all razors, liners and trimmers are disinfected and sanitized before and after every cutting service.

VEGETABLE PARASITIC INFECTIONS

Tinea is the medical term for ringworm, which is caused by vegetable parasites. All forms of ringworm are contagious and can be transmitted from one person to another. The disease is commonly carried by scales or hairs containing fungi. Bathtubs, swimming pools, and unsanitized articles can also be sources of transmission.

Ringworm starts with a small, reddened patch of little blisters. Several such patches may be present. Any ringworm condition should be referred to a physician.

Tinea capitis, ringworm of the scalp, is characterized by red papules, or spots, at the opening of the hair follicles. The patches spread and the hair becomes brittle and lifeless. It breaks off, leaving a stump, or falls from the enlarged open follicles.

Tinea favosa, also known as favus or honeycomb ringworm, is characterized by dry, sulfur-yellow, cuplike crusts on the scalp, called scutula, which have a peculiar odor. Scars from favus are bald patches that may be pink, or white and shiny. It is very contagious and should be referred to a physician.

Ringworm can be minimized by keeping tool implements and work area sanitized with anti-fungal solutions or detergents.

ANIMAL PARASITIC INFECTIONS

Scabies "itch" is a highly contagious, animal parasitic skin disease, caused by the itch mite. Vesicles and pustules can form from the irritation of the parasites or from scratching the affected areas.

Pediculosis capitis is a contagious condition caused by the head louse (animal parasite) infesting the hair of the scalp. As the parasites feed on the scalp, itching occurs and the resultant scratching can cause an infection. The head louse is transmitted from one person to another by contact with infested hats, combs, brushes, or other personal articles. To kill head lice, advise the client to apply larkspur tincture, or other similar medication, to the entire head before retiring. The next morning, the client should shampoo with germicidal soap. Treatment should be repeated as necessary. Never treat a head lice condition in the salon or school. Advise the client when applying shampoos, creams, and lotions that contain *insecticides* (i.e., lindon or larkspur solution) one must use caution. Pregnant women and infants should avoid all insecticide solutions.

The head louse is transmitted from one person to another by contact with infested hats, combs, brushes, or other personal articles.

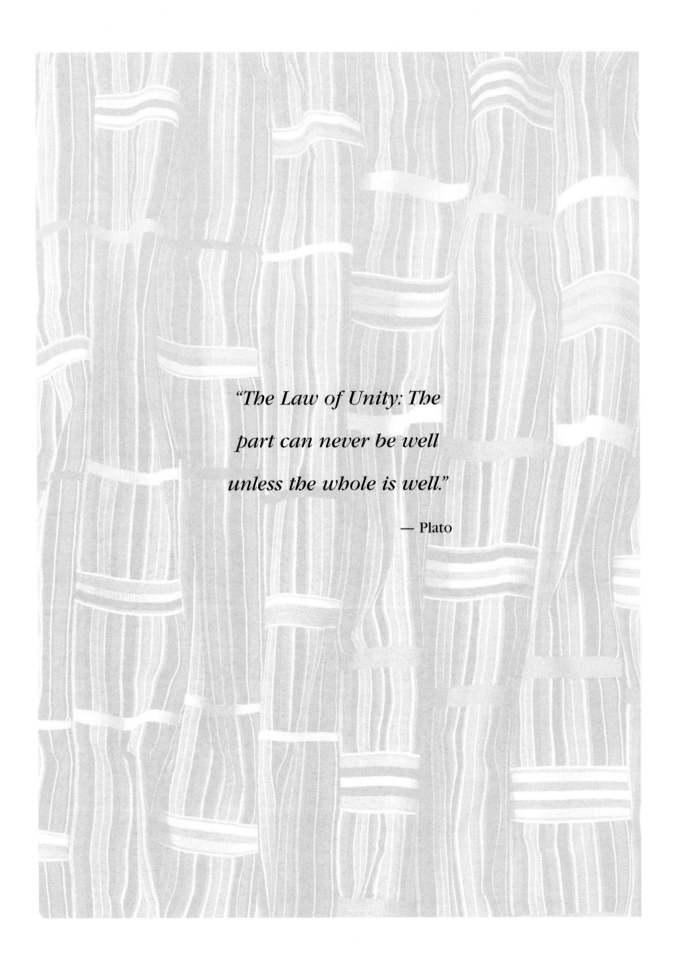

"The Law of Unity: The part can never be well unless the whole is well."

— Plato

CHAPTER 7

Basic Anatomy, Physiology, and Nutrition

KNOWLEDGE BOX

In this chapter you will learn:

1

Structures and functions of the human body

2

Functions of the human cells, tissues, and organs

3

About the body systems

4

The principles of nutrition

INTRODUCTION

A basic understanding of the structure and functions of the human body will help in creating the scientific basis for providing the appropriate service to the client. It is important to understand how the various body systems work as an integrated whole towards wellness.

A healthy functioning body will produce healthy hair. Hair is a part of the whole. As stated earlier, "The part can never be well unless the whole is well." This is particularly true in terms of the interrelated systems of the body. Although the natural hair care specialist may never use the names of the bones, muscles, or nerves in the salon, a general understanding of how they work will increase your proficiency when performing many of the hair care services and braided styles.

SYSTEMS

The groups of organs that work together for the common well-being of the human body are called **systems**. The body is composed of ten systems that sustain the skin, bones, muscles, nerves, blood supply, lungs, waste elimination, stomach, and reproduction. (For further information, see *Milady's Standard Textbook of Cosmetology*, chapter 23.)

Integumentary System — Skin

Blood and lymph supply nourishment to the skin. As they circulate through the skin, the blood and lymph contribute essential materials for growth, nourishment, and repair of the skin, hair, and nails. In the subcutaneous tissue are found networks of arteries and lymphatics that send their smaller branches to hair papillae, hair follicles, and skin glands.[1]

Skeletal System — Bones

Bone structure provides the physical foundation of the body. It is composed of different shaped bones that are connected by movable and

---

[1] Milady's Standard Textbook of Cosmetology, revised edition. Albany, NY: Milady Publishing, 1995, 523.

immovable joints. It shapes and supports the body and protects various internal structures and organs. It also serves to attach muscles and acts as levers to produce body movement.

Muscular System — Muscles

This system shapes and supports the skeleton. Its function is to produce all movements of the body. It consists of more than 500 muscles, large and small, and comprises about 50% of the body weight. Muscles are fibrous tissues. The natural hair care specialist should be concerned with the voluntary muscles of the head, face, neck, arms, and hands. Massage stimulates these voluntary muscles that concern the natural hair care specialist the most.

Nervous System — Nerves

This is one of the most important systems of the body. It controls and coordinates the functions of all other systems and makes them work harmoniously and efficiently. These fine fibers (nerves) cover every square inch of the body. This system is important to the stylist to effectively deliver scalp and facial services. There are sensory, motor, and mixed (sensory and motor fibers) in the nervous system. Sensory nerves conduct impulses or messages from sense organs to the brain, where sensations of touch, cold, heat, sight, hearing, taste, smell, pain, and pressure are experienced. Motor nerves carry impulses from the brain to the muscle to produce movement. Mixed nerves contain both sensory and motor fibers and have the ability to both send and receive messages.

There are sensory, motor, and mixed nerves in the nervous system.

Circulatory System — Blood Supply

The circulatory system is related to maintenance of good health. The vascular system controls the steady circulation of the blood through the body by means of the heart and the blood vessels. The blood-vascular system consists of the heart and blood vessels for the circulation of the blood. The lymph-vascular system consists of lymph glands and vessels.

Endocrine System—Ductless Glands

Glands are specialized organs that vary in size and function. The blood and nerves are intimately connected with the glands. The nervous system controls the functional activities of the glands. The glands have the ability to take certain elements from the blood and convert them into new compounds. The two main sets of glands are **exocrine** or duct glands and **endocrine** or ductless glands. Sweat and oil glands of the skin and intestinal glands belong to the duct glands; secretions of hormones are delivered directly into the bloodstream and come from the ductless glands.

The glands have the ability to take certain elements from the blood and convert them into new compounds.

Excretory System—Organs of Elimination

This includes the kidneys, liver, skin, intestines, and lungs. This system purifies the body by eliminating waste matter. Metabolism of the cells of the body forms various toxic substances which, if retained, might poison the body.

Respiratory System—Lungs

The lungs are spongy tissues composed of microscopic cells that take in air. The tiny air cells are enclosed in a skin-like tissue. Behind this, the capillaries of the vascular system are found. With each respiratory or breathing cycle an exchange of gases takes place. Oxygen is absorbed into the blood while carbon dioxide is expelled during exhalation. Oxygen is more essential to the body than food or water.

Reproductive System—Organs for Reproducing

In females, this system produces the reproductive cells (egg or ova) and includes the uterus, in which the fetus is developed, the fallopian tubes, and ovaries. The male system produces the sperm. Hormones control the well-being of the reproductive system.

Digestive System—Stomach and Intestine

This system changes food into a form that is soluble and readily absorbed by cells to nourish and strengthen the body. Digestion begins in the mouth and is completed in the small intestine. Food that is digested is absorbed into the bloodstream. The complete digestive process of food takes about nine hours. Intense emotions, excitement, and fatigue seriously disturb digestion. On the other hand, happiness and relaxation promote good digestion.

HEALTHY HAIR FROM WITHIN

The quality of the hair and skin are reflections of good or poor physical health.

External and internal sources for hair:
1. Oil—adds luster, pliability, and protection
2. Moisture—keeps hair supple, soft, and hydrated
3. Vitamins and minerals—nourish and fortify
4. Protein—restores and strengthens

Hair is a wonderful indicator of general good health. It is an extension of the skin. The quality of the hair and skin are reflections of good or poor physical health. Although everyone is aware of the need for proper nutrition in order to have a healthy body, most people do not realize that the same holds true for healthy hair. Healthy hair is a product of a healthy body and is mirrored through one's physical and emotional well-being.

Hair gets all its nourishment from the foods we eat. At the very bottom of each hair follicle (a tube-like passage for the hair shaft) is the hair bulb. The papilla is a small blood vessel that feeds the bulb. It is through the papilla that the supply of nourishment reaches the root and the bulb of the hair shaft.

The scalp and hair receive nourishment from the blood stream. It is vital that the circulation of the blood in the body is not restricted or

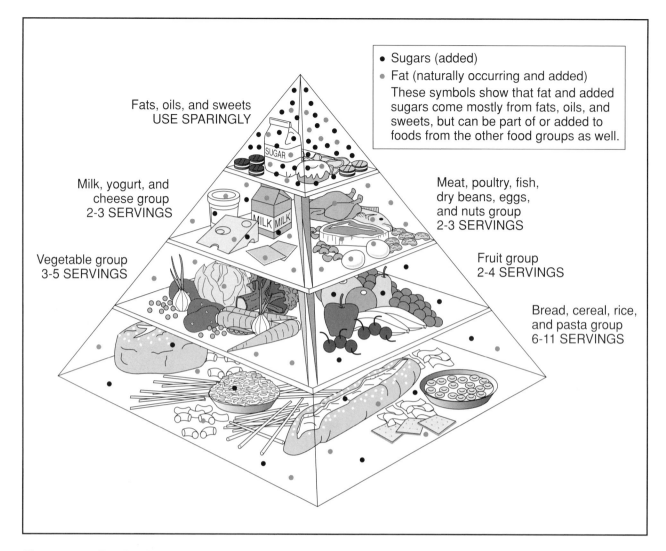

Fats, oils, and sweets
USE SPARINGLY

SUGAR

MILK MILK

- Sugars (added)
- Fat (naturally occurring and added)
  These symbols show that fat and added
  sugars come mostly from fats, oils, and
  sweets, but can be part of or added to
  foods from the other food groups as well.

Milk, yogurt, and
cheese group
2-3 SERVINGS

Meat, poultry, fish,
dry beans, eggs,
and nuts group
2-3 SERVINGS

Vegetable group
3-5 SERVINGS

Fruit group
2-4 SERVINGS

Bread, cereal, rice,
and pasta group
6-11 SERVINGS

Figure 7.1   Food guide pyramid

impaired. A good balanced diet, exercise, and plenty of water will promote the proper properties of the blood and enhance the circulatory system that brings the necessary nutrients to the hair and scalp.

As a natural hair care specialist, you must be aware of the general nutritional value of food. Medically speaking, there is no definitive evidence that proves nutrition is received through topical hair products. All the shampoos, pomades, gels, deep conditioning, and treatment services can only mask dull, weak, dry, broken hair. Healthy growing hair is interconnected with a healthy body. The vitamins, minerals, oils, moisturizing products, and protein substances used topically to protect and groom the hair are necessary, but are secondary to the daily food requirements needed internally to maintain a healthy scalp and hair.

In the Western culture, we eat more food per person than anywhere else in the world. Our diets are filled with sugar, fast foods, and processed foods; meats and dairy products clog our system. As a result of these high demands of refined or processed foods, we expose ourselves to poisonous chemicals and harmful food additives which some studies have found to cause illness and degenerative diseases. Herbicides, pesticides, and fungicides, as well as some fertilizers, when used in large quantities, are poisonous. In the long term they are harmful to the earth and to our bodies. Food additives such as chemical substances to enhance food flavors and preserve "shelf life," colorants, stabilizers, and bleaching agents have doubled in consumption since the 1950s. Natural food additives do exist; however, more than 3,000 synthetic additives are available and are used by more food manufacturers. Growth hormones are additives found in meats and produce. They are used to make plants and animals appear larger and often they reduce the nutritional value. As a rule, we eat more because our bodies require more food to receive the same nutrients. We take in more calories, but are still not sufficiently nourished.

To stay healthy longer, we need to eat the foods our grandparents used to eat. It is safer and nutritionally more valuable to eat whole foods and, whenever possible, organically grown vegetables, fruits, plants, and other food substances.

It is safer and nutritionally more valuable to eat whole foods and organically grown vegetables, fruits, and plants.

What are Whole Foods?

Whole foods are foods prepared or eaten in the natural state. They have not been processed or altered to enhance appearance. Nothing has been added or removed nutritionally. They are the foods that grow closest to the ground.

What are Organic Foods?

Organic foods are foods grown without chemical treatments like herbicides, pesticides, fungicides, synthetic fertilizers, or additives.

Whole food alternative diets can include meat, poultry, and fish, which are usually found at kosher or organic butchers and markets. However, most people that follow a whole food diet, such as vegetarians, do not eat meat, poultry, fish or "flesh foods" of any kind. For the most part, a balanced diet would include lower intake of meats, fats, and processed foods.

> *A balanced diet would include lower intake of meats, fats, and processed foods.*

Foods to avoid or minimize would include the following:

1. *Meats such as beef, pork, and chicken.*

2. *Processed foods (foods with sugar or sugar substitutes).*

3. *White flour and white flour by-products.*

4. *Saturated fats (this increases LDL cholesterol, which can lead to heart disease, cancer, and obesity).*

   - *butter, lard, margarine, some vegetable shortenings*
   - *poultry skin*
   - *beef, pork, bacon, hot dogs, organ meats*
   - *chocolates and white sugar desserts*
   - *corn oil*
   - *coconut oil*
   - *milk and heavy creams*
   - *processed cheeses*

5. *Caffeine and by-products in sodas, teas, and coffee.*

6. *Dairy products. Eggs should be limited to two per week. Some options will be soy cheeses, nonfat cottage cheese, and yogurts.*

7. *Especially avoid the following substances. These substances deplete the body of vital nutrients, vitamins, and minerals, deteriorating the body and increasing the aging process. In excess, these substances can become highly toxic to the body:*

   - *smoking tobacco*
   - *alcohol*
   - *drugs (pharmaceutical and illegal)*

Whole food alternative diets may include the following variety of food substances:

- *grains and beans (which are rich in protein). These are great sources for the essential building blocks for protein: amino acids. They are necessary in the growth and maintenance, repair, hormonal, antibodies and enzyme manufacturing in the body.*

🔊 *Nuts and seeds are high in mono-unsaturated fats. They are excellent in the breakdown of blood cholesterol levels. Second in protein, they are excellent sources of essential fatty acids, which aid in the movement and absorption of vitamins A, D, E, and K. They are instrumental in the hormonal and biochemical processes. They assist in maintaining healthy hair and skin and they provide energy.*

🔊 *Vegetables are low in calories, but high in fiber. You can never have too many vegetables. They are rich in vitamins and minerals. Though fiber has no nutritional value, it is essential to helping the body function properly. Vegetables help break down blood sugar and speed the passage of waste in the intestines, which can reduce some cancers. Dark green leafy vegetables are high in calcium and vitamin B2, needed to strengthen bones and teeth, as well as muscular and nervous system development. Vitamin B2 breaks down fats, carbohydrates, and protein to produce body energy.*

🔊 *Fruits are an excellent source for most vitamins and minerals, carbohydrates in the form of glucose or fruit sugars, and fiber. Whether fresh or dried, fruits are low in fat and high in caloric value. Citrus fruits are high in vitamin C. Other yellow and orange skinned fruits are high in vitamin A.*

Whether fresh or dried, fruits are low in fat and high in caloric value.

🔊 *Seaweeds are great alternatives for sources of protein and vitamins and minerals such as calcium, potassium, sodium, iodine, and iron. Vitamin B12 is vital to producing red blood cells, RNA, and DNA, and maintenance of a healthy nervous system. For vegetarians, seaweeds are an excellent alternative to eggs and other dairy products and can be spread over salads in soups, stews, or pasta, or made into a tea.*

🔊 *Dairy products and non-dairy alternatives are high in cholesterol and should be eaten in moderation. In a vegetarian diet they are eliminated totally. Though they are rich in calcium and vitamin B12, they can be replaced with soy milk and other soy products.*

The following pie chart (Fig 7.2) explains the recommended balance for a whole food diet:

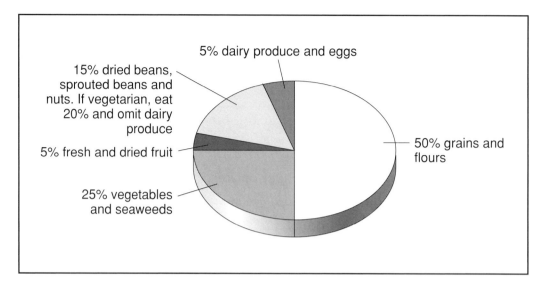

Figure 7.2   The recommended balance for a whole-food diet

The B complex—The Stress Fighter/Balancer

The B complex vitamins provide the body with energy by converting carbohydrates into glucose (sugar), which the body needs to burn in order to produce energy. They are essential in the breaking down of fats and proteins. In addition, the B vitamins are vital in the normal processing of the nervous system and may be the single most important factor for healthy nerves.

One of the richest sources of B complex vitamins is brewer's yeast. Brewer's yeast is also high in protein, B12, selenium, lecithin, chromium, potassium, and eighteen amino acids. It can be added to cereals, yogurt, and other foods, but is most popular in drinks, juices, and shakes. Avoid brewer's yeast if suffering from gout, arthritis, or vaginal yeast infection. Introduce slowly to your diet—one teaspoon daily. The need for B complex increases when the body is under stress or infection. Alcohol and sugars deplete the B complex vitamins. There are supplemental forms of B complex. The lack of B vitamins may be indicated by premature gray hair, falling out or breaking hair, types of baldness, such as alopecia areata, and other skin problems such as eczema and acne.

BAILEY'S HAIR TONIC SHAKE

1 ripe banana

2 to 3 tablespoons of brewer's yeast

8 oz. apple juice, orange juice, or soy milk (vanilla or almond flavor)

1/2 cups of strawberries or ripe pear (optional)

Cut up all fruits and place in an electric blender. Add brewer's yeast and juice. Blend to liquify for 1 minute. Pour into a tall, chilled glass. Enjoy alone as breakfast drink or with cereal, or with whole wheat rolls and nuts. This drink can help boost your energy and keep your hair strong.

NERVE CALMING TONIC

1 oz. oat straw

1 oz. lemon balm

1 qt. water

Oat straw is great as an herbal nerve tonic. It is both relaxing and stimulating to the nervous system. It contains vitamin C and amino acids. Lemon balm is a mild anti-depressant and is cooling to the body.

HEALTHY HAIR AND SCALP DIET

A great "multi" or vegetable tonic can act as a nutritional supplement to a good diet and healthy lifestyle. Always follow recommended daily volume.

Vitamins

A, B complex, B2 (riboflavin), B12, biotin, bioflavonoids, C, D, E, F, K, choline, folic acid, niacin, paba, pantothenic acid, and cysteine. Essential fatty acids are fats or oils not made by the human body yet necessary to the function and maintenance of tissues. Vegetable oils and plant oils, including evening primrose, flaxseed oil, and fish oil such as cod liver oil, are essential fatty acids.

Minerals

Calcium, copper, fluorine, iron, magnesium, phosphorous, beta carotene, potassium, selenium, silica, sodium, sulfur, and zinc.

Vegetables

For a healthy approach to life, you should use this diet to help increase your stamina and allow you to work and be creative.

Asparagus, beans, lentils and sprouts, dark leafy green vegetables (kale, collards), avocadoes, beets, broccoli, garlic, okra, carrots, cabbage, cauliflower, red and green peppers, sea vegetables, kelp, spinach, sweet potatoes, squash, tomatoes, and turnips.

Nuts, Grains, and Seeds

Alfalfa, almonds, brown rice and cereals, flaxseeds, millet, mushrooms, oat brans, pumpkin seeds, sesame seeds, soy beans and products, sunflower seeds, wheat brans, wheat germ, and cereal.

Fruits

Apples, apricots, banana, berries, cranberries, cherries, dates, figs, prunes, grapefruit, red grapes, lemons, papaya, plums, peaches, pears, oranges, raisins, tangerines, variety of melons, mangos, and kiwi.

As a natural hair care specialist, the above recommended diets are also important to your well-being and health. As a role model for a healthy approach to life, you should use this diet to help increase your stamina and allow you to work and be creative. If you adhere to basic nutritional eating habits, you will gain credibility as a professional natural hair care specialist, because it is true that "you are what you eat."

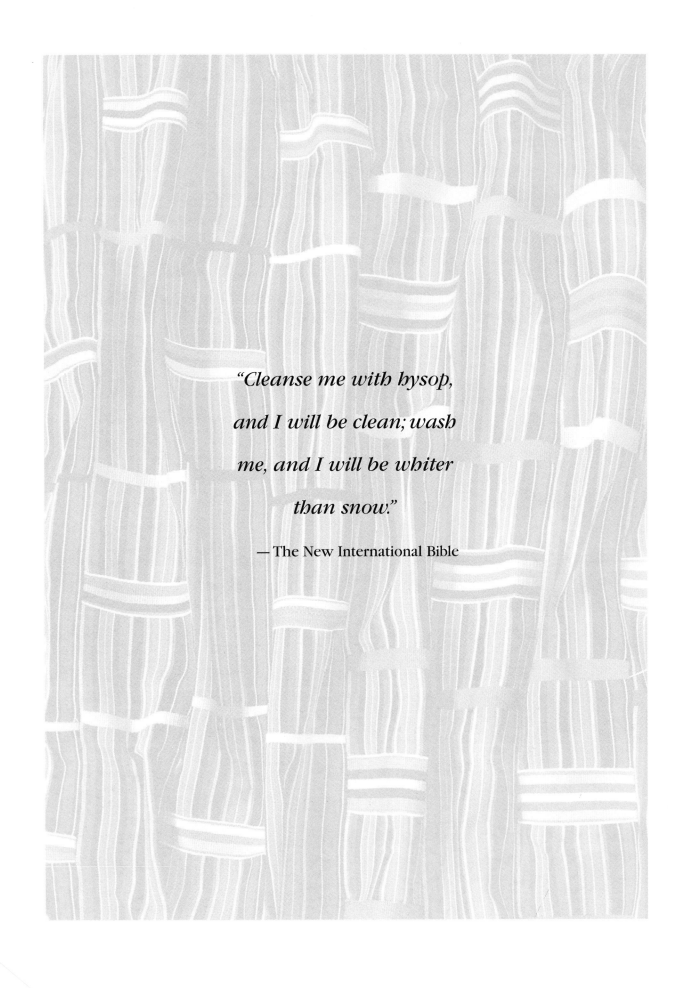

"Cleanse me with hysop,

and I will be clean; wash

me, and I will be whiter

than snow."

— The New International Bible

CHAPTER

Shampoos, Conditioners, Herbal Treatments, and Rinses

KNOWLEDGE BOX

In this chapter you will learn:

1

Nurturing shampoo techniques for textured hair

2

How to shampoo braids

3

How to remove braids before shampooing for touch-ups

4

The different types of shampoos

5

Types of herbal rinses and conditioners

INTRODUCTION

The most precious jewel of the body is the head. It is your crown to the temple, your body. Natural hair care specialists believe that the head is the most spiritually sensitive part of the body. The soft center of the head, called the crown, is sensitive to touch and rhythmic motion. Naturalists believe that the crown area of the head transmits and receives life's energy forces; it is the essence of one's spiritual well-being. This view is not so far-fetched when you recognize that all human functions are engineered from the head. The head protects the brain, which is the command center for what you taste, see, hear, think, and feel. Emotional and physical well-being is rooted in the head.

To the natural hair care specialist, hair is the outer manifestation of the inner being.

In traditional African culture, the head is glorified and adorned because it is treated as the spiritual center of the body. It houses the brain which controls thoughts and emotions. All human functions stem from the head—heartbeat, breathing, digestion, and body movement.

If the head is the conduit of the life's energy force then so is the hair, rooted in the head and extending outward. Hair protects and covers the crown and receives energy. Notice that when you are under physical or emotional stress your hair may shed or break. Such hair loss may result in balding. The Rastafarian culture (mainly in the Caribbean) believes that locked hair is an antenna to God, that locks are spiritually connected to the creator that keeps people emotionally strong and vital.

Therefore, most natural hair care specialists recognize that hair is more than protein and keratin. To the natural hair care specialist, hair is the outer manifestation of the inner being. When hair is properly cleaned and groomed, the mind, body, and spirit are renewed and revived.

During a shampoo treatment, the braid specialist wants to create a relaxing, soothing, seductive experience for the client. It is a treatment that addresses the condition of the hair and scalp as well as the client's well-being. Proper hair care should be a positive transforming experience. Clients come to a salon expecting to be changed for the better. To meet that expectation, hair care must allow for creative sharing and an exchange of energy.

The shampoo experience is the initial service that promotes sharing between the client and stylist. Through the sense of touch, it creates the emotional and physical bond between the two so that ideas and conversation can flow. With every shampoo/treatment experience, the braid stylist must initiate a "healing" or therapeutic process. This healing process begins with the scalp manipulation or massage during the shampoo service. The hands-on healing and soothing shampoo/treatment will transmit energy from the stylist to the client and vice versa. Hands are our creative tools. They are the medium in which our intuitive creative abilities are executed or demonstrated.

There are various healing art forms of massage:

- *reiki*
- *reflexology*
- *Ayurvenda (5,000 years old)*
- *Shiatsu*
- *acupressure*

All forms highlight the full dimensions of the human touch. The Reiki method of healing through massage focuses on the balancing of life force energy and the therapeutic effects of the hands. The natural hair care specialist with skilled and healing hands can affect the body in the same way a doctor uses technical equipment and hands to heal. Through hand manipulation (such as in braiding), the stylist can create a balance of body, mind, and spirit. For clients, looking good makes them feel better and their thoughts and actions are reflected through their outer selves, which says that the beauty was already within them. The stylist only helps the client to release and affirm herself.

With every shampoo/ treatment experience, the braid stylist must initiate a "healing" or therapeutic process.

SHAMPOOING COILED/CURLY HAIR

When cleansing the scalp of the client with naturally curly hair, it is important to comb the hair thoroughly. All tangles must be removed prior to the service in order to prevent the hair from matting or fusing. Hair that has a curly or coil-patterned texture requires a gentle, detangling comb-out before shampooing (see Chapter 9 "Textured Hair is Manageable).

The comb-out will stretch, elongate, and separate the coil-patterned strands, giving the hair a fuller look. If the hair has been recently braided, be aware of debris and loose hair. During the average braided period (two to three months), the natural process of the hair shedding through daily combing or brushing is approximately fifty to 100 strands per day. This is a normal process of wearing braided styles. The longer the client wears a braided style the more the shedding hair will collect during the preshampoo comb-out. It is for this reason that many professional braiders recommend that clients maintain one style for two to three months maximum. After three or four months, braid sediment collects between the scalp base and the extensions. Braid sediment becomes imbedded between the hairs and hardens. It will lead to atrophy (weakening) of the braided strands. An excessive amount of hair comb-out may occur at this point. Hair has a life force energy. If the braids are not removed periodically, the hair will lose its vitality. Atrophy leads to thinning and hair breakage.

Hair becomes weakened and damaged when the braided style is kept improperly and kept in too long.

As professional braiders, we recognize that proper care of the braided style can promote growth and protect the hair and scalp. However, the stylist must educate the client that braids kept in for an excessive amount of time will have an adverse effect on the hair strand. The one comment most often heard in the salon is "the braids took my hair out." This is not correct. Braids do not take the hair out. Hair becomes weakened and damaged when the braided style is kept improperly and kept in too long.

WHY BRAIDS APPEAR TO DAMAGE HAIR

The following is a list of improper braiding techniques and mistakes clients and stylists make that will ultimately weaken hair and cause breakage.

1. An imbalance between the extensions and natural hair. Too often braiders use too much hair in the extension. The exten-

sion material (synthetic/human hair or yarns) should not be too heavy for the natural hair texture. A proportionate amount of extension material must be placed into the braid.

2. *Too much tension. Often braids are too tight and cut off circulation to the scalp, which will eventually cause hair breakage.*

3. *Leaving braid styles and extensions in the hair too long. Braids should not be kept for more than two to three months because the individual strands of hair will become thin and weak.*

4. *Improper shampooing and conditioning of braided styles. Without proper care, oil and cream residue as well as dirt will build up and clog hair follicles. Residue is referred to as braid sediment or debris.*

5. *Chemically treated hair should not be braided right away. The hair should be properly conditioned and braided at least a week or two after a chemical treatment. Ideally, a braided style is best when the hair is all natural. Hair in transition can be braided; however, breakage is unavoidable. When growing out a relaxer, the hair is in transition. The shaft has two textures and at the point where the textures meet, breakage often occurs.*

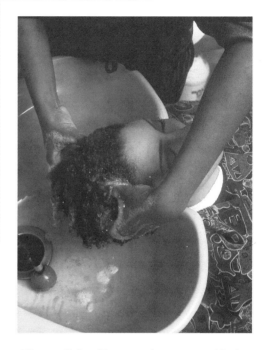

Figure 8.1 Shampooing textured hair.

Shampooing textured hair does not require scrubbing. The object of a shampoo is to effectively remove dirt and oil residue from the scalp. The service should be, as mentioned earlier, soothing and emotionally relaxing. A scrubbing motion can be agitating and harsh (Fig 8.1).

Because of the properties of textured hair, scrubbing can also cause damage. Textured hair is curly, coiled or wire-like. It also tends to be dry, fragile, and easily tangled. It often wraps around itself. If textured hair is scrubbed, it can cause matting and intertwining of the strands and can cause breakage when untangling the hair.

When cleaning textured hair, concentrate on cleaning the entire head in a rhythmic, soothing motion. You want to massage the scalp to circulate the blood as well as to clean the scalp. Good blood flow provides the hair follicles with nutrients hair needs to stay healthy. A relaxing touch and stimulating movements can invigorate the scalp to produce its own natural oil sebum. Sebum is the scalp's natural moisturizer.

With curly hair, the natural oil does not always reach the end of the hair follicle, unlike the case with straight or slightly wavy hair. This limited amount of sebum is why textured hair tends to feel dry and can be brittle. On textured hair the sebum must travel around the twists and bends in the hair and often coats only a small portion of the hair strand. That portion is generally closer to the scalp, leaving the ends of textured hair the least coated. The old wives' tale about brushing your hair from the back to the front (upside down) 100 times a night was popular with clients with straight hair because the blood would rush to the surface of the head and the brushing would bring natural sebum from the scalp to the ends of the strand.

Brushing repeatedly may be productive for straight hair or slightly wavy hair; however, coiled hair/textured hair is too fragile. Bending coils in and out can cause breakage at the curves of the coil where the hair strand is weakest.

When shampooing coiled hair and braided styles, *aim to cleanse the scalp*. The shampoo will remove dirt and oil on the hair when it is rinsed.

When shampooing coiled hair and braided styles, aim to cleanse the scalp.

SHAMPOOING BRAIDS

When shampooing braided styles avoid heavy cream shampoos. No matter how much water you use to rinse cream shampoos a residue will still remain, attracting dirt and weakening the braid.

> ### To avoid or reduce braid sediment do the following:
>
> *1. Avoid heavy cream shampoos that will coat the braid shaft. (These are usually the products that claim to condition and shampoo in one step.)*
>
> *2. Use clear gel shampoos that rinse thoroughly. Dilute if necessary.*

3. Avoid heavy petroleum on braids and scalp.

4. Avoid heavy gels or pomades that attract dust and dirt from the environment.

5. Use a neutralizing or cleansing shampoo, if a cream shampoo has been used in the first washing. This will help strip cream residue. Dilute cream shampoo to avoid braid sediment.

6. Dandruff shampoos are effective for clients with heavy build-up, however they are heavy-cream based. Dandruff shampoos are not recommended for braided or locked hair. They are made with harsh chemicals that strip too much sebum from the scalp. If a client has been using dandruff shampoos, a deep conditioner is required to moisten the hair.

7. Always rinse with hot or tepid water after shampooing. Water spray should be forceful.

8. An acidic rinse (lemon juice, lime, vinegar, and water) can be used to reduce sediments and close cuticles.

9. Squeeze braids downward with a non-pulling motion when rinsing. This may bring sediment that has not been properly rinsed to the surface.

The braid removal service is as important as the service of creating braids.

REMOVING BRAIDS FOR CLEANSING

After extended wear, to give a thorough cleansing and conditioning, the braid style must be removed professionally. Taking out braids is a special skill and can be a separate service which a salon provides. Many clients dread the thought of taking out their own braids. For a client, it is a long and tedious job and if not done properly, can be painful. And like the old adage, "It's a dirty job, but somebody has to do it," so it is with braid extension removal. A salon can provide the service separately and an assistant can be trained for the task.

What is the big deal about removing braids? It is a service that requires skill and practice. The braid removal service is as important as the service of creating braids. The smaller the braids the more time is required to remove them. Also, the more fragile the base of the braid is the more likely it is to be covered with scalp and dirt residue. The average head of medium-sized braids can take one client four to six hours to remove. Each braid must be removed one at a time and combed gently to avoid breakage and scalp irritation. It is a very awkward task for clients to remove their own braids because they cannot position themselves properly to remove them all. Some clients say they feel as though they must be contortionists to remove each braid, often missing a few they cannot reach.

The final phase of removing the braids is detangling and comb-out. It is this part of the removal that can cause clients the most damage because the hair debris is hardened and sebum is crusted at the base of the natural hair. This can cause knots. The knots have to be unraveled gently to have a smooth, free comb-out. When clients attempt to do this task themselves, they become frustrated and anxious. They rush, ripping through the hair, generally using improper tools. In haste, they wash their hair without thoroughly combing it out and cause a worse problem for themselves—hair fusing or matting.

By offering clients a braid removal service, you ensure the optimum care and health of the hair.

Because this task is so great, too many clients delay the process and once again wear braid styles longer than the recommended time. By offering clients a braid removal service, you ensure the optimum care and health of the hair, which is the goal of a professional natural hair care specialist.

Reasons for Providing Braid Removal Service

There are five excellent reasons to provide your clients with a braid removal service:

1. *Ensures safe removal with minimal breakage.*
2. *Saves time.*
3. *Helps maintain proper hair care.*
4. *Allows for partial removal for braid/weave touch-ups.*
5. *Prevents excessive wearing of braid styles.*

How to Remove Braids Professionally

There is a simple method for removing braids professionally, as well as a detangling solution to make the procedure less difficult.

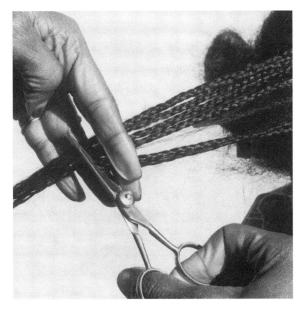

Figure 8.2 Braid removal cutting.

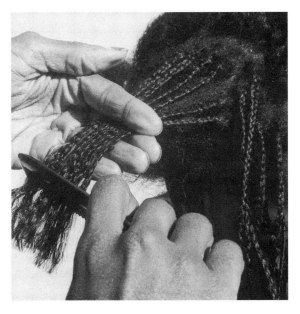

Figure 8.3 Picking motion—combing.

Synthetic and human hair removal may be handled using the following twelve-step technique:

1. *Section hair. The smaller the braid the more sections needed.*

2. *Each section can be handled or divided into subsections, gathering three to four braids at a time.*

3. *Open braids up by cutting off the finished or extended ends. In most cases, look for where the client's natural hair ends and the extension continues, cutting approximately two to three inches below the natural length. Avoid cutting the real hair (Fig 8.2).*

4. *With a small to medium tail or cutting comb, in a picking motion, comb upwards on braid shafts. The motion should be rapid and in a circular pattern. Stay close to the unbraided portion of the braids. Your finger should be positioned on top of the sectioned braids to control the unraveling and support braids to avoid pulling the hair while the comb is working through the braided stitch (Fig 8.3).*

5. *Comb down the braids after several picking motions to unravel the loose ends.*

6. *As the comb gets closer to the base of the scalp, drop the subsections and work on one braid at a time. Comb up the braid shaft until the teeth reach the scalp base, then use the tail end of the comb to open the loop at the base.*

7. *Braid debris must be loosened and removed at this point or once the subsection is unbraided. Do not try to comb all braid debris after the entire head of braids is removed. Remove lint and oil residue section by section to get the best results.*

8. *If braid debris is extremely heavy or crusted, spray a combination of water, cream rinse, and oil to soften hair and detangle. Hair should not be saturated.*

   Detangling Solution

   4 oz. water

   2 tbsp. cream rinse

   3 to 5 drops of natural hair base oil

9. *Once one subsection is completed go to the next subsection and work your way through to the individual braids.*

10. *Use a large-tooth comb to detangle the entire section.*

11. *Twist ends to separate one section from the next.*

12. *Proceed to the next section. Once the entire head is completed, check hair for any residual debris, lint, oil deposits and tangles. Prepare to shampoo.*

SHAMPOOING TECHNIQUES

Proper shampooing technique is essential for both the client's comfort and to maintain healthy hair.

To properly wash and help put the client at ease, the following shampoo techniques should be executed:

1. *Properly drape the client.*

2. *Remove clips, pins, bands, and so on.*

3. *Remove braid debris and excess extended material, if necessary, by combing and detangling with a large-tooth comb.*

4. *Examine scalp and hair for breakage, bald spots, sores, flaking, and general condition.*

5. *If any braid extensions are hanging from thin strands of hair, cut tips of the extension and remove. Avoid pulling to prevent hair from snapping off.*

6. *If there is no need to remove braids, seat the client at the shampoo sink.*

7. *A towel should be draped around the client's neck to absorb excess water from extensions.*

8. *Check water pressure and temperature. Water should be comfortably warm and pressure moderate to strong. Ask the client if the water temperature is comfortable. (It is appropriate to ask clients to close their eyes to avoid splashing in them.)*

9. *Saturate braids or hair extensions. The thicker the braid the more water is needed to penetrate.*

10. *Protect the client's face with a free hand when wetting the hairline with the spray nozzle. Use your thumb and pointer finger to create a shield for the face.*

11. *Once the hair is wet, in the palm of your hand pour a small amount of shampoo. Create an emulsion by rubbing hands and distributing shampoo to the tips of fingers in the scalp.*

12. *Begin at the hairline and apply shampoo to the scalp as well. Apply a moderate amount to the crown of the head, moving and massaging the shampoo toward the back or nape of the head. If necessary, add more shampoo.*

13. *When the shampoo is evenly distributed, work it into a lather with the pads of your fingers.*

14. *As the lather increases, use circular massaging motions and smooth the shampoo downward into the sink. Do not apply much pressure to the braids.*

15. *Pressure applied to the scalp massage should be firm but not painful or intense. Avoid pressure on sensitive or abused areas of the scalp. Do not rub areas where there are open sores or cuts.*

SHAMPOO MASSAGE

A shampoo massage helps to relax the client while stimulating the scalp and promoting healthy hair.

The following ten steps are an effective method of administering a shampoo massage:

1. *With cushion of the finger tips, firmly start at the hairline right above the temple and work the scalp in small circular motions toward the crown of the head. Move around the scalp clockwise with the thumbs around the hairline.*

2. *Move toward the center of the head, palming the head as you massage around the crown.*

3. *Move down toward the ears in a rotary movement. Movements should be small and slow, moving about a 1/2" at a time. If the hair is braided, work into the parts of the braid.*

4. *In some cases, a back and forth movement must be applied to the scalp in order to effectively cleanse the scalp. With braided styles, shampoo the parts between braids to avoid loosening the braid style.*

5. *Moving toward the nape of the neck, lift the client's head gently from the sink with one hand. With the other hand strategically place fingers under and around braids then massage the nape area back and forth.*

6. *Clients should not have to lift their own heads. If the client is relaxed the head should move freely in the shampooers hands.*

7. *This circular shampoo pattern should be repeated at least two times. This will effectively stimulate blood circulation to the scalp and clean the scalp.*

8. *Rinse thoroughly. First rinse the scalp where most of the lather is located. Bring the spray nozzle close to the scalp to give it added pressure and to remove lather from braids. With braided styles, hold the nozzle directly on the braid. Sink water should be cleared of lather to complete the rinse.*

9. *Once water is totally clear, repeat application of shampoo. Shampoo at least two times. The first shampoo just loosens the dirt and oil; the second shampoo actually cleanses. If a third or fourth shampoo is required then the scalp may have a disorder or a problem of excess sebum dandruff. The client may need a special shampoo to address the problem.*

10. *Braid extensions hold water, so gently ring hair downward with both hands to remove excess water before towel drying. Remove all moisture around hairline, forehead, and ears with*

the towel ends. Drape the front of the head with towel, pat gently, and wipe. Hold the hair or braid with the towel a few seconds to squeeze out any excess water. The scalp is now prepared for treatment rinse and conditioning.

CLEANSING AND NURTURING

As a natural hair care professional it is your responsibility to understand and choose the shampoo for varying hair types and conditions. Whether the client's hair is natural or chemically treated, dry, oily, fine, or coarse, there is a shampoo that will best address the needs of the hair type. The market offers literally thousands of shampoos professing to make hair more manageable, bouncy, and "behaving." Others promise to condition the scalp and hair, as well as cleanse. Some even promise to aid highlighting and brightening hair color.

For the natural hair care specialist, less is more. When shampoos promise too many benefits, consumers beware. With the growing industry of natural, less harsh, preservative free or animal-testing free shampoos, options for more wholesome and nurturing products exist. Using shampoos made from herbal extracts and essential oils is effective in creating healthy hair for harmonious hairstyling.

Thousands of shampoo types fill the beauty supply stores. They vary in colors, fragrances, and descriptions for proper hair care. A braid stylist must be aware and knowledgeable about the ingredients that are listed on every product.

Since 1976, the Food and Drug Administration (FDA) requires by law that all hair manufacturers list ingredients which will ensure the safety of the consumer. Labeling regulation requires that ingredients are listed prominently in their decreasing order of prevalence. In other words, the ingredient that is listed first on the label is the most prominent in the product. For example, if water is listed first then that shampoo is largely water with other ingredients included. The last item is the smallest amount contained in the product. If the label is not sufficient in size then a tag containing the ingredients must be attached.

Commercial shampoos are designed to cleanse the hair and scalp; however, too much cleansing agent can strip the natural oil (sebum) which coats the hair. Sebum protects the hair strand and contributes to its luster and manageability. Textured hair is extremely vulnerable because sebum is not evenly distributed on the hair strand and often the hair is dryer and less protected. Oil and moisture have to be replaced manually in order to keep the hair shaft coated. Basic shampoos usually clean well, but they also remove all the natural oils. Textured hair needs mild (or low pH) shampoos that gently cleanse but do not strip the hair of natural oils. Hair braided with extensions require cleansing shampoos that have slightly more cleansing action to remove debris from the braid and scalp.

Textured hair needs mild (or low pH) shampoos that gently cleanse but do not strip the hair of natural oils.

Frequent shampooing of textured, coily, kinky hair will result in extreme dryness and brittleness. The hair must be adequately moisturized after each shampoo. Braided hair should be shampooed about every two to three weeks. Lint, oil, and dust become embedded into the braid and remain on the scalp and must be removed in order to maintain healthy braided styles. So more cleaning shampoos should be used for the first wash. The second or third shampoo, if necessary, should be a milder gel-type conditioning shampoo to moisturize the hair.

For locked hair or natural textured hair, avoid heavy cream shampoos. Heavy creams leave a sticky residue buildup on the hair that attracts more dirt and makes the hair appear dull. Creams become embedded in the hair locks or braids and do not rinse thoroughly. If the cream residue is allowed to build up, it can be harmful to the hair as well. The residue can harden and cause breakage. It can also clog hair follicles and block sebum, which eventually has a drying effect on the hair. Lock sediment actually becomes a part of the lock. Once sediment becomes a part of the lock it is almost impossible to remove without picking apart or weakening the lock.

The Five Classifications of Shampoos

There are five very distinctive classifications of shampoos. There are detergents, low pH shampoos, dandruff shampoos, protein/conditioning shampoos, and herbal/organic shampoos. Basic or commercial shampoos are generally made with synthetic products.

The first ingredient in most shampoos is water, purified or de-ionized. The second most prominent ingredient is the base detergent or base surfactant, which can be used interchangeably to mean the cleansing or "surface active" agent. Surfactants are chemical compounds to create the wetting, emulsifying, dispersing, and liquifying of a shampoo. The third most common agent in shampoos counteracts or complements the negative characteristics of the original base detergent, because the base is generally the harshest chemical.

These are the five basic types of detergent bases that actually clean the hair. They differ in the intensity and removal of hair oil and debris.

Detergents and Understanding pH (Potential Hydrogen)

Detergents are usually high in pH (potential hydrogen) or alkaline, which kills bacteria. However, high alkaline products strip the hair's natural oils. In a shampoo, the pH is only relevant to the strength of the cleansing agent. The ideal pH of hair and skin is usually about 4.5 to 5.5 on the pH scale. The neutral level is 7.0, which is equivalent to pure water containing no minerals (Fig 8-4).

High alkaline products strip the hair's natural oils.

At the optimum pH level, the shampoo should have a low enough acidity to retain the hair's natural fatty acids or sebum which protects the hair shaft and retains moisture.

Essential fatty acids of sebum + Low acidity shampoo (low pH) = Optimum levels of moisture retention in hair and skin.

Some mild detergents (ranging from 4.5 to 6.0 pH) claim not to strip hair oils. But all detergents, whether mild or strong, remove natural oils. It is up to the natural hair care specialist to choose products that minimize this process. The following descriptions can be useful in selecting the appropriate shampoos.

pH — Potential Hydrogen Chart

**The degree of alkalinity or acidity of any water solution.
The pH is a numerical scale
from 0 (very acidic) to 14 (very alkaline).
A pH of 7 is neutral.**

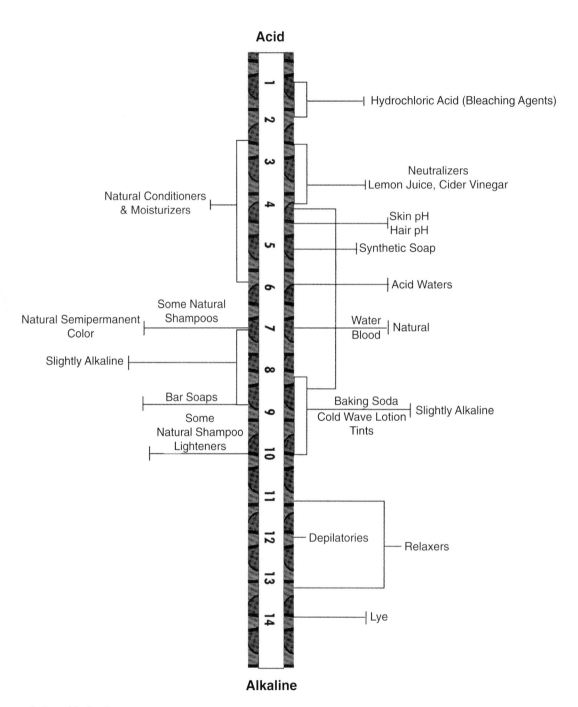

Acid

- Hydrochloric Acid (Bleaching Agents)
- Neutralizers
  Lemon Juice, Cider Vinegar
- Natural Conditioners & Moisturizers
- Skin pH
- Hair pH
- Synthetic Soap
- Acid Waters
- Some Natural Shampoos
- Natural Semipermanent Color
- Water
- Blood
- Natural
- Slightly Alkaline
- Bar Soaps
- Baking Soda
- Cold Wave Lotion
- Tints
- Slightly Alkaline
- Some Natural Shampoo Lighteners
- Depilatories
- Relaxers
- Lye

Alkaline

Figure 8.4 pH chart

Basic Detergent Agents

1. **Anionic (an-eye-on-ik)** This is a high foaming, lots of suds, shampoo. It tends to strip the hair of natural oil. A strong cleansing agent, sodium lauryl sulfate, is used to produce thick lather that rinses well in soft or hard water. Sodium laureth sulfate is milder because it is lower in pH or alkaline and is less drying. According to Dr. Marianne Nelson O'Donoghue, dermatologist and author: "These (anionics) occasionally can be too strong and irritating. This could be because of the pH, or because there is too much detergent action on the hair, which causes too much sebum to be removed."[1]

> ### Other anionics to be aware of in commercial shampoos are:
>   1. *(TEA) Triethanolamine lauryl sulfate*
>   2. *Ammonium laureth sulfate*
>   3. *Lauroyl sarcosine*
>   4. *Cocoyl sarcosine*
>   5. *(TEA) Laureth sulfate*
>   6. *Sodium lauroyl sarcosinate*
>   7. *Sodium cocoyl sarcosinate*
>   8. *Sodium lauroyl isoelthionate*
>   9. *Sodium dioctyl sulfosuccinate*
>   10. *Coconut sulfated monoglycerides*
>   11. *Disodium oleamide sulfosuccinate*
>   12. *Magnesium salt*
>   13. *Potassium salt*

2. **Cationics (cat-eye-on-iks)** These detergents or surfactants are made of quaternary ammonium compounds, or quats. **Quats** have antibacterial characteristics usually found in dandruff shampoos and also found in cleaning disinfectants.

---

[1] O'Donoghue, Marianne Nelson. "Hair Care Products," 1994, 378.

> ### The following are cationics in commercial shampoos:
> 1. Quaternary ammonium
> 2. Benzalkonium chloride
> 3. N-2 ethylaminoformy, methylopyredinium

3. **Monionics (mon-eye-on-iks)** These are detergents that emulsify well and usually have a mild cleansing action. They are gentle to the skin and cause little irritation to the scalp or eyes. However, these products are boosted with **ethonylated compounds** to increase lather. These compounds also increase thickness and solubility. The conditioning agent in these monionics is Sorbitol ester, also known as tweens. They are emulsifiers (or softeners).

> ### Monionics found in commercial shampoos are:
> 1. Diethanolamide
> 2. Polysorbate 20 and 40
> 3. Palmitate
> 4. Monoethanolamide
> 5. Sorbitan laurate
> 6. Stearate
> 7. Ethoxylated fatty alcohols
> 8. Ethoxylated alkyl phenols
> 9. Ethoxylated fatty amines
> 10. Ethoxylated fatty amides

4. **Ampholytes or amphoterics** These detergents cling to the hair making it appear more manageable. They contain germicidal or antiseptic characteristics and are often used in baby shampoos because there is no irritation to the eyes or skin. They are the mildest of detergents and claim not to strip the natural oils from the hair and scalp because they have a gentle moisturizing effect.

According to Dr. Wesley S. Wilborn, dermatologist and author of articles about African-American hair growth disorders, "Shampoos that contain anionic agents are particularly drying to the hair. An example is sodium *laureyl* sulfate. The sodium *laureth* sulfate shampoos are not as harsh, but (Negroid) African hair needs shampoos that contain humectants and milder cleansing agents, such as amphoteris and nonionic blends."[2]

> ***These are the ampholytes found in most commercial products:***
> *1. Sodium lauraminopropionate*
> *2. Triethanolmine Laureaminopropionate (TEA)*
> *3. Cocamide betaine*
> *4. Amphoteric 1 through 20*

The natural hair care specialist must realize that detergents are found in all products whether they claim to be natural or not. Even in health food stores, one out of ten cosmetic shampoos claiming to be organic and herbal had one or more sulfactants listed. This means that in order for most products to be user-friendly and have a longer shelf-life, many chemicals must be used.

You are not limited to commercial products. It depends on the specialists' philosophy as to how natural their products must be. The goal, however, is for the natural hair care specialists to be in balance with their environments and the demands of their businesses. Find products that can satisfy both.

The natural hair care specialist must realize that detergents are found in all products.

Low pH Shampoos

The commercial low pH shampoos are designed for the consumer with dry, brittle, damaged hair. They contain milder cleansing agents that do not strip all natural sebum. However, in most cases, **pH balanced** products are difficult to measure (no one walks around with litmus paper to test for the acidity of a product). "Shampoos claiming to be pH balanced may be

---

[2] Wilborn, Dr. Wesley. "Disorders of Hair Growth in African-Americans," 1994, 391.

more of a marketing strategy than a real actuality," notes Aubrey Hampton, author of *Natural Organic Hair & Skin.*[3] No matter what the product promises to do, the normal pH of hair and skin is quickly restored after regular washing. "Any alleged value to the pH balanced protection lasts about as long as it takes the product to wash down the drain," says Hampton. In addition, research shows that a shampoo having a low pH does not necessarily mean that a product is nurturing to the hair.

On a pH chart, lemon juice and hydrogen peroxide rate as having a low pH or low acidity. However, used when applying permanent color, hydrogen peroxide can dry and damage hair. Diluted lemon juice, on the other hand, is an excellent conditioner for removing shampoo residue and debris from braided and locked hair. It too has a low pH, but it helps to maintain the essential fatty acids and sebum that protect the hair and scalp. Pure lemon juice can irritate the scalp and dry the hair.

Natural hair care specialists must educate themselves on the different products that claim to offer pH balanced ingredients. These products can leave the hair and scalp dry and itchy because of the additives, preservatives, and fragrances.

For textured hair, the naturalist should consider products that offer the most natural ingredients with essential fatty acids (essential organic oils). Essential fatty acids cannot be produced. The human body must be supplied through diet and application of organic oils found in seeds, extract of vegetables, and animal fats. These fatty acids are labeled as "essential" because they are so necessary for life. The hair and scalp needs the following organic oils for normal growth and natural luster.

> *Research shows that a shampoo having a low pH does not necessarily mean that a product is nurturing to the hair.*

The following natural oils with essential fatty acids have excellent moisture-retaining properties and are high in Vitamin F and minerals:

1. *rosemary oil*
2. *sage oil*

---

[3] Hampton, Aubrey. Natural Organic Hair and Skin Care. Tampa, Florida: Organica Press, 1984, 39.

3. evening primrose oil

4. glycerin

5. shea butter

6. linseed oil

7. flaxseed oil

8. cod liver oil

Linoleic acid, linolenic acid and arachidonic acid are all essential fatty acids.

Dandruff Shampoos

Dandruff shampoos contain **active ingredients** that help control scalp flaking or scalp disorders like seborrhea dermatitis or psoriasis. Most anti-dandruff shampoos are basic detergent shampoos with harsh, drying ingredients. They treat the problem of the scalp but also remove too much of the natural oils that protect the hair.

Most anti-dandruff shampoos are basic detergent shampoos with harsh, drying ingredients.

The following are some of the ingredients added to dandruff shampoos that address and treat scalp flaking, seborrhea and psoriasis:

1. tar

2. selenium disulfide (most effective and harsh)

3. zinc pyrithione (least drying)

4. salicylic acid

5. zulfur

6. kekoconazole

Most of these ingredients are added to moisturizing shampoos (particularly zinc pyrithione, tar, salicylic acid) so you can shampoo more frequently without stripping the scalp. A study provided by the University of Pennsylvania adequately demonstrated that there is "an increased epidermal cell turnover in seborrheic dermatitis" when using shampoos with these additives.[4]

For textured hair types, these anti-dandruff and anti-seborrheic shampoos, such as selenium sulfide shampoos, are extremely damaging. The natural hair care specialist must take extra care when serving the client with these scalp conditions.

For textured hair types, anti-dandruff and anti-seborrheic shampoos are extremely damaging.

As an alternative, the following procedure can be used to avoid the harsh effects of these additives. This procedure can be done on all hair types.

1. *For the first shampoo, put the medicated shampoo in an applicator bottle with a small nozzle top. Part the wet hair in 1/2" sections and apply the product until the entire scalp is covered.*
2. *With small circular motion, massage the scalp until the lather covers the scalp. Avoid vigorous motions to limit the shampoo to the scalp.*
3. *Shampoo thoroughly and allow the lather to remain on the scalp for three to four minutes so that the active ingredients can work.*
4. *Rinse; apply second application.*
5. *For the third shampoo, use a mild moisturizing, herbal, or conditioning shampoo.*

Aesthetic Shampoos

Protein, Conditioning, and Moisturizing Additives These are shampoos with little to no stripping effect on natural hair oils. They are more gentle than most shampoos but are not thorough cleansers. Regardless of what the label indicates, these shampoos do not penetrate the hair shaft.

They are usually composed of some of the milder anionic, monionic, and amphoteric surfactants. Hydrolyzed animal proteins are added to the basic shampoo to address split ends and damaged cuticles and to increase elasticity. But most protein shampoos coat the shaft, giving the hair strand

---

[4] O'Donoghue, Marianne Nelson. "Hair Care Products," 1994, 379.

more bulk or body. Many esthetic shampoos have conditioners and moisturizers to make the hair more manageable.

These shampoos are often designed so that they do not rinse out thoroughly. Instead, they leave a deposit of film to add some moisture back into the hair. The additive fills in the gaps on the hair cuticle. The cuticle of the hair shaft becomes damaged due to heavy chemical use or from direct heat from pressing and excessive blow drying. It is also affected by chlorine and sun exposure.

You will also find that many of these milder shampoos are designed with sunscreen agents to protect color-treated or permed hair from the damaging sun rays. They can be useful products to protect **virgin hair** from harmful environmental elements and do not strip natural oils. But they are also so mild that they have very little cleansing action.

Shampoos that contain honey or honey shampoos act as emollients to seal in moisture and contain humectants or moisture retainers. These aesthetic shampoos work effectively as products used on the second or third shampoo to detangle and soften textured hair.

Herbal or Organic Shampoos

Herbal or organic shampoos offer the best alternative to commercial shampoo products.

For the natural hair care specialist, herbal or organic shampoos offer the best alternative to commercial shampoo products. After an extensive study comparing natural extracts to their synthetic copy, Aubrey Hampton says, "There was invariably a difference between the synthetic and the natural extract. The difference was that the body responded differently to the real substance than to the synthetic substance. Using the synthetic copy of a natural extract on the skin or hair in cosmetic formulas gave me an inferior product every time from every standpoint. Pure vegetable glycerine, for example, is a thicker, richer, and a far better emollient than synthetic propylene glycol (the petro-chemical replacement usually found in moisturizers). The synthetic chemical is usually substituted for the natural extract because manufaturers believe the scientific hype 'you can't tell the difference...' What they can't measure, however, is the body's response to natural substances.

It is believed that natural substances reinforce the cosmos within you, and synthetic substances create chaos. The chaos referred to is the disharmony and imbalance within one's self—that would also include unleashing emotional, physical, and spiritual selves.

The use of herbs in hair products is our way of staying connected to the earth and its importance to our existence. Herbs are the tools we use to repair our bodies and explore our consciousness or spirituality, as well as helping us to remain a part of the earth's total ecology."[5]

As David Hoffman explains: "The realm of plants provides everything our body needs for a balanced and integrated existence. However, we are more than just a body. We also have consciousness, which brings other factors onto the stage. We not only have to take our animal body into consideration, but also our emotions, our minds, and our spiritual nature. Harmony is no longer simply a matter of right diet or even right herbs, but also a matter or right feelings, thoughts, lifestyle, attunement, actions—harmony of right relationships to our world and ourselves."[6]

Using healthy, affirming products is very important in developing a relationship with your client.

As mentioned previously in Chapter 3, cultivating harmony is a vital part of the natural hair care service. Using healthy, affirming products is very important in developing a relationship with your client. The all-natural hair client will have greater results with organic or herbal products. These clients who have made the conscious decision to wear their hair naturally need to have quality products to groom, protect, and complement the body's healing ability.

Herbal, organic products do not mask the problem like many commerical products do. Instead, they enhance the hair and scalp and increase their ability to heal. With natural products, there is no quick fix solution.

Natural products can be altered or designed to address each client's needs. Hebal rinses can be added to commercial shampoos to enhance and assist in the cleansing and moisturizing process. Herbal shampoos and rinses should be designed to address the specific needs of the client. It is an easy procedure to follow—several drops of an herbal infusion or herb extract are

---

[5] Hoffman, David. <u>The New Holistic Herbal.</u> New York: Barnes & Noble Books, 1990, 75.
[6] Ibid.

added to the product. With this understanding, the natural hair care specialist can create a new "recipe" that will address particular hair care needs. There is no immediate gratification when working with nature. You will see the improvements in the hair over the long term. The stylist must make the client aware of the long term effect of organic products on the body and in their lives.

It is useful to know that some synthetic products can also be helpful in the servicing of natural hair. The stylist must be conscious of the long term effects of that product as well. Natural and synthetic products can be high in toxicity and can cause some reaction on the skin. Read and understand all product labels before using the product. It will allow you to educate yourself and the client.

What is an Herbal Shampoo?
A real herbal or organic shampoo is not made with detergents or surfactants. The more basic herbal shampoos contain castile soap or black soap. Soaps were used before detergent shampoos were marketed in the 1930s. Soaps can be mixed with a variety of excellent herbal infusions that will address the needs of individual clients. A moisturizing or emollient herb as well as herbs that add an aromatic quality to the product should be a major component of a natural shampoo. There are also optional ingredients for enhancing color, stimulating growth, reducing hair thinning, and solving dandruff problems.

A moisturizing or emollient herb should be a major component of a natural shampoo.

When looking for products that offer natural ingredients, there are several questions the natural hair care stylist should ask. The stylist will need more than one kind of shampoo. Consider the many different hair types, overall conditions, required results, as well as finished look for braids, extensions or locks and weaves of your many clients.

You should ask yourself the following questions before using a new product:

1. *What are the main ingredients the product contains? (Remember: The first few ingredients listed on the label are more prevalent in the product than any other ingredient.)*

2. *Does the product contain synthetic or natural ingredients that should be avoided? Beware of the toxicity in all products.*

3. *Does the product have enough of the desired ingredients that will benefit the client's hair and scalp needs? Many manufacturers add natural ingredients to attract the consumer but do not add enough to have any beneficial effect on the hair.*

4. *Do benefits of the product outweigh the disadvantages? Most natural products still contain a number of preservatives, surfactants, and fillers to enhance color or fragrance.*

5. *Is the packaging much more attractive than the product itself? Some of the highly commercial products look more attractive, serious, and medicinal than they really are. Do not be fooled by packaging; read the labels carefully.*

TIPS

Some naturalists often use black soap or castile soap based shampoo.

Herbal Rinses and Conditioning Treatments Shampooing is the first step in the regime. The second or third step of the natural hair care regime (depending on whether the hair is dry or oily) is the use of natural herbal rinses or tonics. Herbal rinses are excellent preconditioners or "hair food" that nourish the hair and scalp.

NOTES

Herbs are living substances growing on the planet in order to feed earth and all humans. Traditionally, African philosophies believe that living forms of life have energy. They respond to light, air, heat, water, electricity, and music, and have growth cycles. Therefore, they are alive and have a "life force." This life force is the purpose or root of all self healing and body nourishment. As we move away from the natural state of herbs, the less life energy the substance maintains, the less healing and nurturing properties it has, and the less beneficial it will be to your well-being.

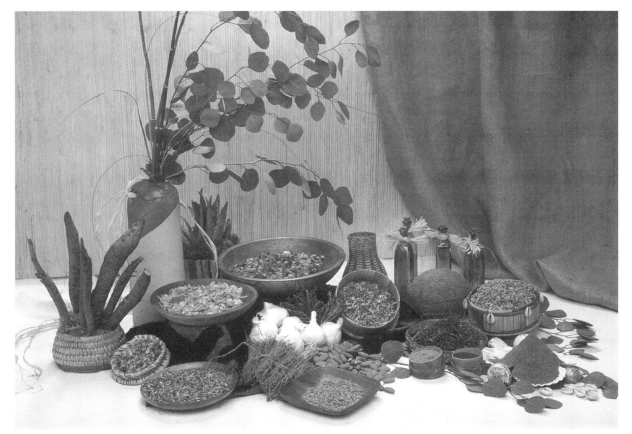

Figure 8.5 Herbs for the natural hair care specialist

The earth has produced natural botanical medicines that address every symptom the body can experience. The body has a natural healing ability and herbs enhance that process. The vitamins, minerals, and nurturing properties of the herbs can condition, stimulate, and strengthen textured hair.

HERBS AND OILS

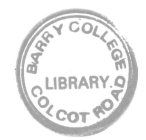

Natural Hair Care Applications

This list of botanicals is presented to give the natural hair care specialist working knowledge of how to enhance any service you provide to your clients (Fig 8.5). Whether the specialist adds several drops of an essential oil or extract to a commercial product, or is inspired to create a customized blend of conditioning treatments, the innate properties of these botanicals can enhance the quality and condition of the hair and scalp.

As the public demands more environmentally safe products and "back-to-basics" hair care, hair care specialists will be required to know more about alternative chemical-free products and treatments.

These oils can be used in combination or singularly. It is important that oil treatment be applied warm because the oils become thinner when heated and penetrate the hair shaft and scalp more easily.

Oily Scalp

Peppermint	Eucalyptus
Bergamot	Lemongrass
Witch hazel	Rosemary
Basil	Thyme
Yarrow	

Antiseptic

Thyme	Camphor
Balsam Tolu and Peru	Citrus rinses
Chamomile	Eucalyptus
Comfrey	Myrrh
Lemongrass	Sage
Tea tree oil	Lemon juice

Moisturizer

Almond oil	Avocado oil
Chamomile	Comfrey
Basil	Aloe Vera
Cocoa butter	Shea butter
Glycerine	Lanolin
Lecithin	Apricot oil
Castor oil	Jojoba

Hair Loss

Jojoba oil	Rosemary
Nettle	Thyme
Calendula	Coltsfoot
Horsetail	Sage
Kelp	Rose hip seed oil

Hair Growth

Camphor	Rose hip seed oil
Coltsfoot	Horsetail
Nettle	Kelp
Sage	Rosemary
Dandelion	Jaborandi
Lavendar	Thyme
Aloe Vera	Burdock root
Basil	Avocado oil

Scalp Soothers

Chamomile	Camphor
Comfrey	Jasmine
Aloe Vera	Almond oil
Olive oil	Avocado
Sage	Eucalyptus

Anti-Dandruff

Sage	Olive oil
Rosemary	Goldenseal
Horsetail	Hysop
Calendula	Evening primrose
Tea tree oil	Garlic
Jojoba	Patchouli
Neroli oil	Burdock root

Cell Rejuvenation

Echinacea	Calendula
Comfrey	Aloe
Lavender	Papaya
Rose hip seed oil	

Softener

Lavender	Papaya
Rose hip seed oil	Castor oil
Ginseng	Evening primrose
Coltsfoot	Coconut oil
Rosemary	Sandalwood
Jojoba oil	Borage
Avocado	

Conditioner

Jojoba oil	Kelp
Sage	Almond oil
Burdock root	Evening primrose
Thyme	Rosemary
Nettle	Eucalyptus
Lavender	

Astringent

Lemon juice	Yarrow
Peppermint	Nettle
Rosemary	Sage
Sandalwood	Chamomile
Witch hazel	Lavender
Sage	Balsams
Tea tree oil	

The following section is a list of herbals, botanicals, and oils that can enhance the hair and scalp. Use the list as a guide to choosing the herbs that are best for the individual needs of the client. When reading labels, look for the herbs that are nourishing to the total being.

External Applications of Herbs

N O T E S

Many of the herbs listed include information about the scalp and skin. One must understand that the scalp is skin. The health of the scalp determines the health of hair. When the body is stressed, the scalp is the barometer of its health status.

Aloe Vera

For centuries, the aloe plant has been known for its first-aid value. This "medicine" plant cleans and relieves burns, soothes sunburns, and heals minor cuts and abrasions. It is also used on cold sores. It helps in the promotion of new growth of living cells, can help stop stinging pain, reduce infection and scarring. It contains antibiotic properties (polysaccharides), healing hormones, and dozens of amino acids, enzymes, vitamins and minerals such as calcium, potassium, sodium, manganese, magnesium, iron, lecithin and zinc. The gel within the plant is 95% water filled with properties that stimulate the scalp. The gel is excellent for African locks and is useful during the locking service to nurture hair. It can be added to creams and lotion to use directly on the scalp as a moisturizer. It softens and has a soothing, cool, refreshing quality. The gel may have a mild drying effect when used alone, but acts as a great emollient when vitamin E oil is added.

For best results, use fresh aloe gel. The plant is very easy to care for. Remove its thick leaf and slice in the middle. Scrape the gel from the leaf with a spoon and add to any moisturizing treatment for grooming gels or lotions for locks. Dermatologists have used aloe to treat oily scalp and dandruff. Pure gel from the plant is often used during the cultivation of locks to accelerate the locking process.

Almond Oil

Almond oil is often used as a base oil in treatments, lotions, and creams. It acts as an emollient and moisturizer and is soothing to the scalp. It contains protein, copper, zinc, vitamin E, essential fatty acids (stearic, lauric, oleic and linoleic) which have excellent moisture retaining properties similar to natural sebum. Apricot and peach oils can often be substituted because they, too, are great moisturizers.

Avocado

Avocado is an essential oil used to stimulate hair growth. Pulp from this edible fruit can be used in facial and scalp packs for concentrated and penetrating treatments. It is filled with vitamins A, D, and E, potassium, sulfur, chlorine, fatty acids and amino acids. Glycolic improves circulation with massages. It also moistens and softens.

Balsam of Peru/Balsam of Tolu

This is a very special aromatic flower and bark. It contains mild antiseptic properties and kills parasites (such as ringworm) and their eggs. This balsam aids in the regeneration of skin cells and is used in shampoos, conditioners, and perfumes for its fragrance. It is a disinfectant and stimulant and contains benzoic and cinnamic acid esters, which are natural preservatives.

Basil

Basil is considered a sacred herb in India, and in certain parts of the country it is dedicated to the Gods. It is called the love herb because of its aromatic qualities. This herb can be used in rinses or tonics to bring shine and luster to the hair. For dark hair, it can be mixed with rosemary as a rinse; for blonde or light brown hair, it can be added to chamomile rinses. Basil stimulates hair growth and reduces snarls and tangles when it is mixed with oil of lavender as a grooming aid. Some Arabian women use this mixture as a hair perfume. In general, the fragrance stimulates and invigorates the senses, promoting growth. Basil contains high amounts of calcium, phosphorous, iron, magnesium, vitamins A, D, and B2.

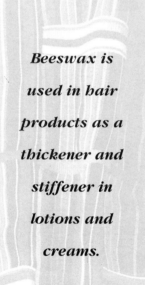

Beeswax is used in hair products as a thickener and stiffener in lotions and creams.

Beeswax

Derived from honeycomb, beeswax is used in hair products as a thickener and stiffener in lotions and creams. It is also used as an emulsifier to keep products from separating. It contains 71% fatty acid esters and is used on locks to keep them in a cylindrical shape. However, beeswax also leaves a very heavy coating and attracts dirt and debris from the environment when used as a grooming agent for locks.

Bergamot (also Beebalm)

Bergamot herb is an essential oil used in hair products, toilet water, colognes, floral and heavy perfumes, as well as soaps for its scent. Because it is so fragrant, it is a soothing aromatic that helps clear the head and relieve tension. Bergamot oil (derived from fruit) is used on the scalp as a preparation for greasy hair. When used in a rinse, the herb can stimulate the scalp. It builds resiliency in hair after it has been damaged. As a facial treatment ingredient, it may cause skin sensitivities or redness. It is a remedy for such skin problems as acne, boils, cold sores, eczema, and oily complexions.

Burdock Root

Burdock taken internally is a great blood purifier. It helps to promote kidney function and nourishes poor functioning pituitary glands (responsible for hormone balance). Externally, burdock root is extremely cleansing and soothing to skin problems such as acne, canker sores, dandruff, and eczema. When used as a rinse, it will address flaking, scaly scalp problems and will restore tones. It helps dark hair tones maintain their color. It can strengthen follicles that have been stressed from poor grooming. Nutrients found in burdock are large amounts of vitamin C and iron, 12% protein, and 70% carbohydrate. It also contains some vitamins A and B complex, vitamin E, PABA, sulfur and small amounts of silicon copper, iodine, and zinc.

Calendula (Marigold)

Calendula has a mild astringent quality. When flowers are used in an infusion, it can be effective in washing cold sores and irritated skin. It cleans and soothes cuts, abrasions, eczema, and acne as well as scalp disorders such as dandruff. It also helps to heal and relieve minor pain. Calendula is also effective in rejuvenating skin cells. As a moisturizer, it can soften hair and scalp. When used as a vinegar rinse, calendula can enhance natural highlights in dark brown and blond hair. It contains a large amount of phosphorous and some vitamin A and C.

Chamomile (gold and blue)

Chamomile is one of the most popular herbs in the world. Its aromatic essence of apple is sweet and wonderful for potpourris. Internally, chamomile acts as a sedative and relaxes the nerves and upset stomach. It soothes and calms without harmful side effects and induces sleep. Externally, it is excellent for relieving eczema and skin inflammation. In shampoos and rinses, it cleanses as well as moisturizes to soften hair gently. When combined with a neutral henna as an infusion and rinse it can give dark hair golden highlights. It has a penetrating quality so it is great to use as a facial or herbal hair treatment. Chamomile stimulates the natural hormone thyroxine, which influences and rejuvenates the texture of the skin and hair. Chamomile contains calcium, magnesium, potassium, iron manganese, zinc, and vitamin A.

Chamomile acts as a sedative and relaxes the nerves and upset stomach

Coltsfoot

Coltsfoot contains large amounts of cystine and silica which are excellent for the hair—both cystine and silica are important foods for the hair root. Cystine is an essential amino acid which is a protein (keratin) derivative of the hair. The purpose of the cystine is to restore and repair protein in the hair. Coltsfoot helps prevent hair loss due to overprocessing and over manipulation. As an extract added to a hot oil treatment, rinses, or tonics, coltsfoot renews and stimulates growth. The sulfur in the herbal extract absorbs into the scalp and aids in correcting dry scalp or seborrhea (oily scalp) and hair loss due to stress. It contains high levels of vitamin A and C, potassium, vitamin D, zinc, B12, B6, silica, and cystine.

Castor Oil

Comfrey contains a natural hormone called allantoin, which helps to strengthen bones and healthy skin cells.

Castor oil beans (seeds) have been found in Egyptian tombs that were more than 4,000 years old. Used internally, it is a laxative. Externally, it is a moisturizer as a base oil to moisten or soften skin. It is often found in transparent soap and shampoos for dry hair. Castor oil is rich in essential fatty acids and can be used to nourish hair and scalp. It can be used as an emulsifier in ointments, grooming products, creams, and lotions. When using castor oil as a base, other oils must not be toxic in order to avoid scalp irritation or laxative reaction.

Comfrey

Comfrey is a powerful healing herb and an excellent emollient. As a healing agent, comfrey is an astringent which helps clean and destroy bacteria. It can aid in healing cuts, abrasions, and sores. It softens and soothes skin and scalp, which is vital to regeneration of cells and tissue. Comfrey contains a natural hormone called **allantoin**, which helps to strengthen bones and healthy skin cells. It can be used in an herbal rinse and tonic because of its amino acid and protein content; it is useful for dry, damaged hair and overprocessed hair. It can retard hair loss.

Cocoa Butter

Cocoa butter is a derivative of the cocoa plant which gives us chocolate. This thick, fatty oil has the fragrance of chocolate. In the form of cocoa butter it is an excellent lubricant and skin softener. It is often used as a base to mix with other vegetable oils and coconut oil to protect the scalp from flaking.

Dandelion

Dandelion is an excellent stimulant to promote circulation; it is also a mild astringent which cleans and aids in healing. It is a great source of protein which helps to strengthen the hair. It can help regenerate skin cells and soothe an over-sensitive scalp. As a refreshing rinse or tonic, it can invigorate a dull scalp.

Echinacea

Echinacea is considered the "king of blood purifiers." It stimulates the body's ability to fight against infection and builds up the immune response. It regenerates skin cells to promote healing. When used topically, the antibiotic echinacea neutralizes healing. Internally, it is a natural cleanser which benefits the skin. It contains vitamins A, E, and C, iron, copper, sulfur, and potassium.

Eucalyptus

Eucalyptus is a very common herb in Australia where over 500 species comprise more than three-quarters of the vegetation on the continent. Eucalyptus oil has an extremely antiseptic and antibacterial quality. The active germicide agents it contains prevent infection. It has a very aromatic and stimulating scent. It cools and soothes the scalp and is usually found in products that address dandruff and flaking scalp conditions. This is an effective herb for shampoos because of its cleansing properties, but it must be used in small amounts to avoid irritation and toxicity.

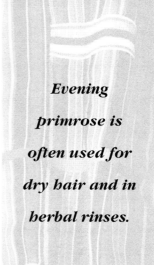

Evening primrose is often used for dry hair and in herbal rinses.

Evening Primrose Oil

Evening primrose oil is an excellent moisturizer and softener. It is high in fatty acids, which is good for many body functions as well as for hair follicles. It is used in creams and lotions to allow a product to safely coat and protect the hair strand and scalp. This coating is not greasy and increases absorption when mixed with other oils. Evening primrose is often used for dry hair and in herbal rinses. It must be used in small amounts to avoid sensitivity or irritation.

Fennel

Fennel is a very sweet aromatic herb that tastes like licorice. It is excellent for herbal steams and rinses, and facial and/or scalp treatments. It opens and medicates pores. It is an effective cleansing and rejuvenating herb for skin cells. It is often found in creams and lotions and contains sulfur, potassium, and sodium.

Frankincense

Frankincense is known as one of the gifts offered by the Three Wise Men to the baby Jesus. It is extremely aromatic and used mostly in incense. When used as an oil it can be a stimulant with a warm, soothing quality. It removes dead skin cells and relieves flaking from severe dermatitis; it promotes healing of minor cuts and burns.

Garlic

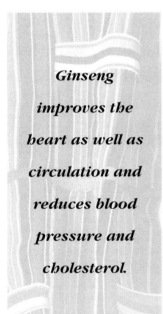

Ginseng improves the heart as well as circulation and reduces blood pressure and cholesterol.

Garlic is a natural antibiotic. Its strange odor destroys bacteria, fungi, and yeast. It stimulates cell growth and rejuvenates the healing process. It is high in essential fatty acids which protect and strengthen the hair strand. The sulfur compounds reduce microrganisms and repair damaged hair follicles. Garlic is excellent for treating dermatitis and skin inflammation. Garlic contains vitamins A and C, selenium, sulfur, calcium, manganese, iron, copper, and vitamin B. It is high in potassium and zinc.

Ginseng

Ginseng is known as the king of herbs. Internally, ginseng stimulates the entire body by increasing resistance. Ginseng improves the heart as well as circulation and reduces blood pressure and cholesterol. Externally, its silica content strengthens and repairs protein bonds in hair and it soothes the scalp as well as stimulates growth. It can reduce scalp flaking. Natural glycerides contained in ginseng moisten and soften hair. Ginseng contains vitamins A and E, thiamine, riboflavin, B12, niacin, calcium, iron, phosphorus, sodium, silicon, potassium, manganese, magnesium, sulfur, and tin.

Goldenseal

Goldenseal is used primarily by the Cherokee Native Americans in a mixture to stain their faces and dye clothing. As used by the Native Americans, it is a natural insect repellent. Cosmetically, goldenseal is an astringent, cleaning tonic used to reduce bacteria, fungi, and cold or canker sores. It has anti-dandruff properties and is excellent when used in shampoos, rinses, and tonics. Goldenseal contains vitamins A, C, E, F, and B complex, calcium, copper, potassium, phosphorus, manganese, iron, zinc, and sodium.

Henna

Henna is an herb generally made into a powder. In a clay form it has been used in Egypt for more than 4,000 years to color hair, palms of hands, feet and nails. It is an excellent source for coloring oily hair. As a colorant, the powdered herb coats the hair with a thin film staining and leaving hues or highlights and shine. Commercial henna colors vary in shades from neutral for brightening to deep blues and blacks that cover grey hair. Paprika can be mixed with henna as a hair rinse to color hair reddish bronze. The film residue henna leaves on thin hair gives hair the appearance of thickness and adds body. Henna has an astringent quality that can control oily scalp. However, it can be very drying to dry hair types. Neutral henna is often used in shampoo and rinses to neutralize pH and bring hair back to a stable pH state.

Hops

Hops is best known for its sedative quality. When used topically it has a calming and soothing affect on the scalp. It is used as a mild antiseptic and astringent. It has a very strong aroma and helps reduce stress. It is excellent when used as a rinse or hot oil treatment to reduce dermatitis. As a colorant, it can give hair a brown hue. As an infusion with chamomile, it reduces swelling.

Hibiscus acts as an emollient for moisturizing and softening most hair types.

Honeysuckle

Honeysuckle is known for its aromatic sedative fragrance. As a hot oil treatment, it soothes and calms the scalp. It is often used in shampoos and soap because of its cleaning properties. Topically, it is an emollient, moisturizer, and softener.

Hibiscus

Hibiscus is a beautiful flower native to North America and West Indies that can be used as a gentle colorant to give the hair a reddish tone when used in a rinse. Hibiscus must be used repeatedly in order to intensify color. Hibiscus can be mixed with other herbs to add a reddish hue. Also, hibiscus acts as an emollient for moisturizing and softening most hair types.

Horsetail

Horsetail is said to heal ulcers and stop bleeding wounds when used externally. Typically, horsetail oil or extract is mixed with coltsfoot to stimulate the scalp for hair growth and repair. It is rich in silicon and cystine acid found in the sulfur compound of hair protein, which is essential to creating a healthy hair infrastructure. Shampoos and conditioners that offer proteins mixed with sulfur-containing amino acids (silica or cystine) are said to be excellent products to promote growth and stimulate follicles to prevent hair loss. Horsetail in shampoo curtails dandruff because it is a cleansing astringent that increases scalp circulation, reducing seborrhea conditions. As a hair rinse (horsetail, coltsfoot, rosemary, and sage combined) it promotes the general health of hair and scalp. Use horsetail after chemical damage or episodes of alopecia. Rich in silicon and selenium (which helps the scalp but can be drying to hair) it contains vitamin E, pantothenic acid, PABA, copper manganese, sodium, cobalt, iron, and iodine.

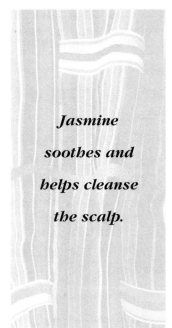

Jasmine soothes and helps cleanse the scalp.

Jaborandi

Jaborandi is considered an essential oil that stimulates hair growth. As an herbal rinse or tonic, it opens pores and extracts impurities. As a steam or bath, jaborandi removes excess water from skin tissue. It is a mild antiseptic and can induce perspiration.

Jasmine

Jasmine is most famous for its aromatic, sultry fragrance. In shampoos, creams, and lotions, it is primarily used as an aromatic because of its variety of fragrances. Topically, jasmine soothes and helps cleanse the scalp. Jasmine oil can be used in rinses or hot oil treatments, or simply massaged into the scalp to sedate and calm. The olfactory reaction produces a feeling of euphoria and optimism and is used as an antidepressant, according to researchers. Jasmine as a tea, or in some German wines, is said to be an aphrodisiac. It is generally non-irritating and can be used on sensitive skin. It is claimed to rejuvenate aging skin by improving elasticity, and reduces inflammation and itching.

Jojoba

Jojoba is known as the liquid wax. It is an extract from the cactus-like plant. It is used by Native Americans for cooking and hair and body grooming. It has an extensive history of promoting hair growth because it is extremely rich in nutrients that restore, protect, and moisturize the hair. It is a vegetable based oil that mixes well with other herbal extracts, while resisting rancidity and extending shelf life. It is an expensive oil said to replace sebum. Hot oil treatments and conditioners with this oil will address hair loss problems due to extreme dryness. This "liquid gold" also aids oily scalps by removing embedded sebum, making the scalp less acidic. It contains amino acid, silica, B complex, vitamin E, chromium, iodine, copper, and zinc.

Kelp

Kelp is an algae derived from the sea, rivers, and ponds. It is a very popular food that is high in nutritional value. Kelp is filled with vitamins A, C, F, and B complex, calcium, and sulfur. The sulfur contains silicon (a strengthener). Kelp stimulates metabolism and nourishes hair. It contains thirty minerals such as cobalt, nickel, silver and titanium. The plant extract contains phosphorous, iron, sodium, potassium, chlorine, copper, zinc, manganese, and small amounts of lecithin.

Lavender stimulates the scalp while acting as a calming agent.

Lavender

Lavender is cultivated throughout the world and is a native to the Mediterranean. There are more than twenty-eight species cultivated. Because of its popular aromatic fragrance, it is often found in perfumes. As an essential oil, it is an antibiotic, antiseptic, detoxifier, and also an anti-depressant (fragrance uplifts the emotions). It is useful in healing burns and cuts because it rejuvenates skin cells. Lavender stimulates the scalp while acting as a calming agent.

Lemon Grass

This botanical has its origin in Central America and Sri Lanka. Lemon grass is an essential oil used to normalize oil production for dry and oily scalp conditions. Lemon grass is very fragrant, light, and antiseptic. In a hot oil treatment for both dry and oily scalp, lemon grass is very effective. It is an excellent source of vitamin A, which helps to heal and soothe dry skin. It can be used for all skin types and can be found in most perfumes, deodorizers and antifungal products.

Lemon Juice

It is native to Southern Europe and North Africa, and is cultivated world-wide. Lemon is a very strong astringent, antibiotic, and disinfectant. It is very aromatic with a sharp, clean but light fragrance. In a rinse, it restores acid mantle of the hair and scalp (natural pH) and stimulates the scalp. It can aid as a bleaching agent or highlighter. But because it rids hair of stale smells and odors, it can tingle or irritate the scalp if it is not diluted properly. It is full of vitamin C. When diluted and used as a rinse, it can soften debris in locked hair. Lemon can also be used during the locking process to lift cuticles, and help coils to spiral.

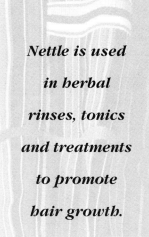

Nettle is used in herbal rinses, tonics and treatments to promote hair growth.

Myrrh

This ancient botanical is at least 2,000 years old. In ancient Egypt myrrh was often used in the embalming process and valued spiritually for its perfume. Its medicinal uses include antiseptics, astringents, and disinfectants. Myrrh has antifungal properties and is known to kill ringworm. It can also be a preservative in other oil mixtures. Myrrh is commonly used in toothpaste, chewing gum, and mouth washes. Because of its strong fragrance, it is relaxing and soothing to the nervous system. On the scalp, myrrh soothes, dries, and fortifies hair.

Neroli Oil

Neroli oil is derived from the orange blossom and has a delicate scent. Fragrance is said to be an antidepressant that counteracts shock and fatigue, nervousness, and insomnia. Neroli oil is also an antibacterial agent and antiseptic to the skin. On the scalp its regenerative properties promote the new growth of skin cells. It also reduces inflammation and soothes irritated skin.

Nettle

Nettle is commonly used in hair and skin products because of its stimulating effect on circulation. Rich in silicon, which helps to restore protein, nettle is used in herbal rinses, tonics and treatments to promote hair growth. Often it is used with horsetail, coltsfoot, rosemary, and sage—other hair growing botanicals. Rich in chlorophyl, which gives nettle its green color, it provides essential trace minerals needed for healthy hair and skin. It is an important food for the hair root and follicle. Nettle is mildly astringent and a natural cleanser and tonic. As a rinse, it softens and soothes dry skin; it can also neutralize an overly acidic scalp mantle. It contains vitamins A, C, E, F, and P, calcium, sulfur, sodium, copper, manganese, chromium, and zinc and is high in protein.

Olive Oil

Internationally known, the olive branch is a symbol of peace. The olive tree is one of the oldest trees on record. Olive oil from the olive itself is an excellent emollient used in all types of cosmetics, shampoos, soaps, lotions and creams. It is an excellent base oil to mix with other essential oils, rinses and tonics. It is very effective as a hot oil treatment for dry hair and scalp when mixed with vitamin E and coconut oil. Lemon juice and olive oils make a soothing rinse. Olive oil and chamomile can be used as an infusion to moisturize and soften dry hair.

Peppermint

Peppermint (as well as other mints such as bergamot, spearmint, pennyroyal, and pineapple mint) are excellent for the digestive system. Peppermint relieves cramps, nausea, hangovers, and motion sickness. It is also an excellent decongestant. Even when used topically, peppermint as a hot oil treatment opens breathing passages. Menthol in herbal mints are stimulants to the scalp and have a cooling effect. It can improve dry, lifeless hair. With its antiseptic properties it cleans and removes embedded oils and can be wonderfully refreshing when added to vinegar rinses or herbal rinses. It can leave the scalp feeling tingly and restores balance to an oily scalp. Avoid using peppermint on clients during pregnancy because of its anti-spasmodic properties. It contains vitamin A and C, magnesium, potassium, inositol, niacin, copper, iodine, silicon, iron, and sulfur.

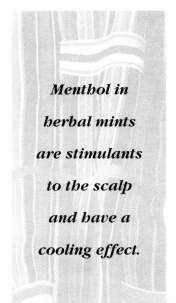

Menthol in herbal mints are stimulants to the scalp and have a cooling effect.

Parsley

Used as a hair rinse, parsley is excellent for all hair types. It is especially soothing and healing in cases of eczema and psoriasis. It is highly nutritious for the hair. It is often found in shampoos, perfumes, soaps and other natural cosmetics. It is an excellent hot oil treatment for an overall healthy scalp. It contains high levels of iron, chlorophyl, vitamins A and C, sodium, copper thiamine, riboflavin, and small amounts of silicon, sulfur, calcium, and cobalt.

Patchouli Oil

Patchouli oil is an essential oil that is an anti-inflammatory, antibacterial, antifungal antiseptic. It cleans as it helps to remove flaking in eczema and dandruff. Patchouli oil is very aromatic, often used in perfumes, and can be found in mouthwashes.

Rose

The rose is native to the Middle East and is cultivated worldwide. It symbolizes love and passion, which is one reason why it is used so often in perfumes, oils, and soaps. The petal from the flower is a mild astringent; as a rinse, such as rosewater, it is great for a dry, flaky scalp.

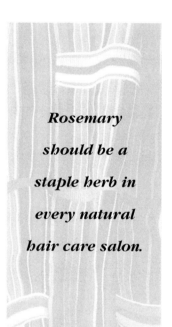

Rosemary should be a staple herb in every natural hair care salon.

Rose Hip

Rose hip refers to the fruit of the rose plant and is an excellent source for vitamin C, more so than oranges. It is very nourishing to the scalp and helps fight infections.

Rose Hip Seed Oil

This oil is derived from the seed. It is potent and concentrated with vitamin C. It is also high in fatty acids (similar to the properties of horsetail and coltsfoot) and aids in the production of collagen-protein, which is helpful to the skin because it rejuvenates skin cells. Rose hip seed oil has large amounts of silicon—an amino acid which is necessary for protein metabolism. It adds elasticity and strength to the hair strand. When mixed with other oils, it helps to prevent hair loss and balding. Rose oil is generally very expensive. It is effective when treating different types of alopecia. It contains vitamins A, E, D, P and C, as well as high levels of vitamin B complex, some iron, calcium, potassium, and sulfur.

Rosemary

Rosemary should be a staple herb in every natural hair care salon. Whether used as an herbal rinse or an oil, rosemary has a long history as a strong stimulant for hair growth. It feeds the root of the hair. It makes a great conditioner for all hair types. Rosemary oil has a very aromatic fragrance that stimulates the olfactory senses. As a mild astringent, mixed with lavender, basils, and nettle, it cleanses and aids in the healing process. It is known as the herb of remembrance—good for the memory.

Sea Salt

Sea salt can be used as a rinse and can be useful in the locking process. It changes the acid mantle of the hair. It affects the pH factor of the hair, opens the hair cuticles and gives the strand a rough, dry touch. The open cuticle is layered and allows the hair to coil around itself easily. Sea salt as a rinse has a healing effect but may be irritating to a dry, sensitive scalp.

Shea Butter

African shea butter, as it is also known, comes from the nuts or seeds of the Butyrosperum Parkii Kotschy tree. This light, non-greasy butter is an excellent pomade for dry, damaged hair. It is often found in shampoos and natural products as a moisturizer and softener. The plant oil or fat has the ability to protect the skin and hair from ultraviolet rays that cause sunburn and dry out the hair. Shea butter is very effective because it is low in acidity and high in fat and waxy substances which protect and coat. In its natural state, vegetarians cook with it as a substitute for dairy butter. In West and Central Africa, shea butter is used to fry foods, as well as for a cream and moisturizer for the skin and hair.

Shea butter is very effective because it is low in acidity and high in fat and waxy substances which protect and coat.

Tea Tree Oil

Tea tree oil has been used by the Aborigines for hundreds of years as a gentle but highly effective antifungal disinfectant. The volatile oils in tea tree oil create a powerful soothing and cleansing agent. When used in shampoos, rinses, and conditioners, tea tree oil stimulates and irrigates the scalp. The oil is similar to peppermint and eucalyptus and should be warm when applied but cool after it is rinsed. It is a great additive for shampoos to fight dandruff and flaking.

Thyme

Thyme is a powerful herbal antiseptic with healing properties. It can be antifungal as well as a rinse to remove crabs and lice. It is excellent as a general tonic for all hair types. As a stimulant, thyme can accelerate skin cell growth because it contains sulfur and silicon. It is often used in a mixture of herbs with similar or compound properties such as sage, lavender, comfrey, rosemary, and peppermint.

Witch Hazel

Witch hazel extract is distilled from the bark of common trees. It is commonly found in hair and skin products as a mild astringent. It is popular in after-shave products because it helps stop external bleeding. It is used as a massage liquid and body lotion. In hair rinses, witch hazel is a cleansing astringent that leaves volatile oils and amino acids which condition and stimulate the hair and scalp. Witch hazel contains 15% alcohol and should not be used regularly on a dry scalp.

As a stimulant, thyme can accelerate skin cell growth because it contains sulfur and silicon.

Add an emollient to witch hazel rinses to moisturize and counteract the alcohol's drying action. Witch hazel helps fight dandruff and soothe inflamed skin. It closes pores, tones skin, and refreshes. It is often used to cleanse the scalp between touch-ups while wearing braided styles. It can be used with cotton balls or swabs between parts to freshen the scalp. Rub lightly and avoid saturation to the hair.

Ylang-Ylang

Ylang-ylang essential oil is often found in cosmetics to groom the hair. It is a mild stimulant which helps blood circulation in the scalp. It has a mild menthol component that cools and helps regulate the sebaceous gland. Very aromatic, it relaxes and soothes nervous energy and acts as an emollient on dry hair. Because of its cleansing and detoxing properties, it makes a great additive in shampoos and rinses. Ylang-ylang is good for all hair and skin types, especially overactive sebaceous glands or seborrhea.

CONDITIONING

Rinses and Tonics

After a mild shampoo, the hair still needs a conditioning agent to give it manageability, strength, and luster and to further cleanse the hair or scalp. Rinses are usually a mixture of distilled water with a mild acid, herbal, or oil base designed to benefit the hair in a particular way.

Rinses can be customized to address any hair problem. What rinses do, generally, is provide protective coats or nutrients to the hair.

Types of Hair Rinses

<u>Acid Rinses</u>—These neutralize or restore the pH balance (acid mantle) to the hair. They remove soap residue and braid and lock debris. They remove build-up from heavy cream shampoos. Hair coated with debris and soap scum can break and become dull so acid rinses are great for locked hair. They also seal in nutrients by closing the cuticle layers of the hair shaft.

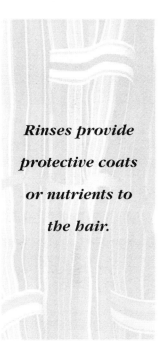

Rinses provide protective coats or nutrients to the hair.

Acid rinses can be made of citric acids, such as lemon juice, lime juice, orange juice, grapefruit juice, and cactus juice. Acidic aids are apple cider vinegar or distilled white vinegar. A tartaric acid can be wine, champagne or beer (but they can leave an odor that must be rinsed out). Lactic acid is derived from a lactose or sugar of milk. Beer can be added to shampoo or used as a rinse to add luster, soften hair, and reduce residue.

Refreshing Lemon Rinse

All hair types

2 whole lemons, juiced and strained

1 quart distilled water

2 to 3 drops of lemon oil or lemongrass oil

Place a medium size bowl or a perming bib to catch the rinse. Apply rinse until the solution becomes cloudy. Use as a final rinse after shampooing and conditioning to close hair cuticle. Do not rinse out.

Citrus Lightener

4 Lemons

4 Limes

2 to 3 drops of lemon extract

With the aid of the summer sun this rinse will add luster, brighten and lighten locks. This mixture will dry hair—always re-moisturize with a hot oil treatment.

Lemon Rinse for Locks

For normal to dry hair

5 oz. or 5 whole lemons, juiced and strained

2 oz. cool distilled water

5 to 10 drops of rosemary oil or extract

2 to 5 drops of almond oil, if hair is very dry

This lemon rinse will cleanse, stimulate and leave a little moisture. Use as a final rinse after a hot oil treatment. This rinse accelerates the coiling process. Catch rinse in a basin, pouring and re-pouring through the hair.

Apple Cider Vinegar Rinse

1 quart cool distilled water or spring water

4 tablespoons of apple cider vinegar

6 to 8 drops of lemon oil or lemongrass extract

This acid based rinse restores, removes shampoo residue, and removes dead skin cells to prevent dandruff, and cleanses and closes hair cuticles. It must be rinsed out well.

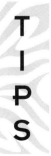

TIPS

Dried Kombu seaweed can be boiled into a rinse or added to shampoo to restore hair color and shine.

Cream Rinses—These are temporary conditioning commercial products. Cream rinses are applied after the shampoo to soften, detangle and add luster to the hair. Most are very fragrant, having a creamy or pearlized appearance.

The cream appearance is aesthetic but can cause problems if used improperly. Cream rinses are great to use when detangling textured hair after a shampoo. Wet, coily hair is very fragile. Cream rinses coat the hair and allow the large-tooth comb to glide through the hair. By using a cream rinse the hair actually becomes temporarily manageable. To avoid a heavy build-up of these topical cream rinses, dilute the cream rinse. It will still be effective.

Light Detangler

4 oz. of distilled water or spring water

2 teaspoons of cream rinse

5 drops of sweet almond oil or any base oil

Shake well before using. Put solution in a spray bottle. Before combing out textured hair, spray solution on each individual section of hair. Comb to detangle starting at the ends first.

Heavy cream rinses should be avoided when conditioning hair with braid extensions or locks. The heavy coating never rinses out thoroughly; a thin film will remain and become embedded in the braid or lock. It leaves the hair dull and unsightly with clumps of cream residue. Avoid cream rinses for clients with human hair extensions. Cream rinses will soften the entire braid and cause it to slip away from the base. However, some stylists use the cream rinse to give the braid extension a fuller hair effect. If you must use a cream rinse, apply it to the ends of the braid extension only. Though cream rinses appear to solve many hair problems, use them selectively and in moderation on all hair types. They can be harmful to the hair over a period of time, because of residue and coating build-up.

Never use creams or waxy products on locks. This creates sediment or residue which can lead to breakage and unattractive deposits.

Herbal Rinses—The best hair conditioners on the market do not only enhance the aesthetic beauty of hair and make it easier to manage, they are also nutritional for the hair and scalp. They can help eliminate hair problems or correct the source of the problem.

Natural hair care specialists approach hair conditioning from two perspectives: internal replenishing and external treatment. Internal replenishing means to restore and replace the necessary nutrients the body needs to survive and maintain health, with a strong understanding of nutrition. As a service, the specialist wants to replenish and help the client maintain healthy hair and scalp. It is not enough to camouflage the problem. It is necessary to keep the hair in its most healthy and natural state with a variety of conditioning agents. Detergents and synthetic shampoos often strip the natural oils and properties that protect hair. Herbal rinses restore natural hair properties.

"Natural" products are usually safe, but some may be toxic or cause scalp sensitivity. A patch test will enable you to determine whether any products used will affect the client with any negative results.

External uses of herbal rinses can aid in coloring, enhancing, and conditioning hair while replenishing essential oils, vitamins, and minerals. They can stimulate the vitality of hair to help it grow.

Some herbal rinses are used as treatments for severe hair problems; others are more fragrant and cosmetic. But all give back something beneficial to the hair.

Herbal Strengthening Infusion or "Power House" Infusion

1 quart distilled water or spring water

1 tablespoon rosemary

1 tablespoon nettle

1 tablespoon burdock root

1 tablespoon sage

4 to 8 drops of tea tree oil, peppermint oil, or lavender oil

This herbal infusion is great on all hair types and is externally beneficial to locked hair styles. The herbs have nutrients that fortify and stimulate growth. The oils cleanse and purify, removing dead skin cells. Both tea tree oil and peppermint oil are mentholated and tingle the scalp. Lavender oil has astringent and soothing qualities.

To prepare an infusion, use a non-metal electric pot to boil water. Thoroughly mix herbs in a separate bowl. Pour boiled water over the herbs and cover. Do not allow the herbs to boil. Boiling herbs destroys their properties. Steeping herbs extracts the active ingredients. Steep for twenty to thirty minutes—the longer the better. (The client can be serviced with a hot oil treatment or deep conditioner while awaiting the infusion).

Strain the herbs from the pot or bowl. Add 1 1/2 cups of cool water to make the solution comfortable. Add oils, shake and pour cooled mixture over clean wet hair. Gently rub into scalp and down the hair shaft. Use an infusion as a final rinse on dry hair and locks.

This type of infusion can be sprayed through the hair daily to correct or resolve hair and scalp problems. It is great for thinning, breaking or over-processed hair and is excellent for use on braided and locked hair. As a spray, the solution is easier to use. Hair will only absorb what it needs. You can massage the solution and rub it down the hair shaft. Spray locks directly.

Botanical Colors and Herbal Rinse

In natural hair care treatments, chemically altering colorants are forbidden by most state regulations. Check and follow your state regulations in reference to color or dyes.

Conditioners that enhance hair color are available for the naturalist to use. They are not reactive or structurally altering chemicals but are clays, powders, and/or liquid mixtures that highlight, condition and embellish the natural hue of the hair.

For thousands of years, henna has been used in many parts of the world. Eygpt, parts of West Africa, Arabia, Persia and India, to name a few, have used henna to add highlights to the hair and as a cosmetic stain to the palms of the hands, nails, and soles of the feet. The wonderful thing about henna is that it is non-toxic to the scalp and skin. Pure henna compounds are generally soothing and do not irritate the scalp. Hennas are offered in a variety of semi-permanent hair stains.

NOTES

Personally, I prefer to call them "stain" instead of color because true colorants require a chemical reaction to the hair shaft. Henna does not penetrate the shaft; instead the hue accumulates on the outside of the hair shaft.

Henna stains can be mixed with an herbal rinse to condition and highlight. For a more effective shade of color, a henna can be mixed with boiling water, made into a paste and applied directly to the hair. Adding heat or moisture aids the processing time. Staining the hair with henna may take several applications because the colors are subtle and, in some cases, unpredictable in intensity. The average time frame for a staining service is 1 to 1 1/2 hours.

Henna works best on oily hair or on dry hair that gets oily by the end of the day. It also aids in the removal of dead skin cells or dandruff flaking. When using henna on dry hair, always re-moisturize as a final step.

Hues range from neutral, which has no hue, to hues such as marigold, copper, dark brown, blue, and black. The botanical powders also give thickness and body to hair (refer to "Henna" section on page 145).

There are other botanicals that can be used to enhance color. Herbs such as hibiscus, for example, add red tones to hair; chamomile adds a gold hue to light colored hair; burdock and black walnut darken hair. Staining or highlighting hair takes longer to see true results, but the process is safer and non-abrasive to the scalp.

Instant Conditioners—These are quick, temporary treatments. They generally coat the hair in order to make it more manageable and give sheen and fullness to the hair. Instant conditioners are useful to protect the hair from the sun and blow drying. Some contain vitamins and botanicals. These ingredients can be good for the hair but are often combined with waxes and detergents that can damage hair. Therefore, most instant conditioners have only cosmetic value. They coat and soften hair but provide very little deep conditioner to repair damaged hair.

Instant conditioners coat and soften hair but provide very little deep conditioner to repair damaged hair.

Protein Conditioners—Protein conditioners usually contain **polymers**, which are small molecular combinations of any twenty-three amino acids. These amino acids are what make up the keratin-protein in hair and skin. They are used to recondition and strengthen hair strands. Protein conditioners are more concentrated and are meant to stay on the hair for at least twenty minutes, which may include a heat or steam application. Heat helps to break down the protein molecule and allows it to pass through the cuticle of the hair, directly into the cortex. Deep protein conditioners can help close split ends. They increase the elasticity of the hair and reduce breakage. They also improve porosity as well as soften and lubricate the hair strand.

Avoid using protein conditioners or deep conditioners on braid extensions or locks. Again, these products come with heavy creams or lotions and leave a film on the braided or locked style.

NOTES

Moisturizers—Moisturizing conditioners are formulated to penetrate the hair. They have many of the same properties as instant conditioners; however, with the application of heat or steam, these conditioners are more effective and longer lasting. Deep conditioning with these products requires a fifteen- to twenty-minute application.

Many moisturizers contain quaternary ammonium compounds (quats). Some moisturizers have an antibacterial action (often found in dandruff shampoos). Quats are also used as an environmental disinfectant. Quats are included in the moisturizing solution of conditioners because they counteract the drying effects of anionic (harsh) detergents. Quats, such as stearatkonium chloride, enable the cream moisturizer to adhere to the hair strand and protect it longer than instant conditioners could.

N O T E S

Avoid using these type of cream conditioners on locked or braided styles, because they leave a residue and make the hair dull. This can lead to breakage, also.

Moisturizers contain humectants that attract and seal water to the hair shaft. Oils protect, add shine, and seal in water, allowing for easy combing and styling. Moisturizers can generally be used without any problems; however, some active ingredients can cause acne on the forehead and stimulate scalp disorders common among African-Americans, such as seborrheic dermatitis.

According to some dermatologists, some ingredients that may aggravate seborrheic dermatitis, or induce inflammation or follicullitis are lanolin, castor oil, wheat germ oil, and soy bean oil.

The most effective conditioning moisturizers offer natural vegetable glycerine, instead of **propylene glycol**—a synthetic which can be irritating to skin and mucous membranes when found in spray form. According to Aubrey Hampton, author of *Natural Organic Hair and Skin Care*, the vegetable glycerine is "extremely superior." It was found that pure vegetable glycerine is a thicker, richer, and far better emollient than the chemical replacement. Still, manufacturers prefer the synthetic product over the natural extract because they believe that you cannot tell the difference.

Petrolatum (such as Vaseline™) and mineral oils are also emollient conditioners, but they can cause irritation to the skin and actually dry the skin. They absorb poorly and inhibit the occurrence of natural moisturizing.

<u>Natural Moisturizers</u>—Sebum is the most natural lubricant (emollient) that the body produces. It protects and softens the hair and scalp. Essential fatty acids are nature's replacement for sebum. **Essential fatty acids** is the chemical term for organic oils found in vegetable or amino fats. They are absorbed into the skin to soften and lubricate. The body cannot manufacture these organic oils or fats. They must be supplied through diet and external application. Hair loss, dullness, and drying due to water loss result when the body is deficient in essential fatty acids.

Fatty acids act as natural agents, sealants, or barrier substances which leave a thin coat on the surface of the hair and skin and protect the hair and skin from drying conditions. They help the body conserve water (moisture) on the skin.

Hair loss, dullness, and drying due to water loss result when the body is deficient in essential fatty acids.

Some moisturizers (or humectants) commonly listed on product labels are:

propylene glycol (synthetic)

glycerol (natural or synthetic)

glycerine (natural or synthetic)

sorbitol (natural)

The unsaturated compounds of organic oils found in products include:

linoleic acid

linolenic acid

arachidonic acid

oleic acid

> ### *Saturated compounds include:*
> *pametic acid*
>
> *stearic acid*

These organic oils have excellent moisture retention properties. They are effective nurturing emollients that have high penetration on the hair and scalp. However, these organic herbal oils and extracts should be added to base oils to enhance their therapeutic value.

Many of the essential oils in the pure form are very concentrated. Most must be diluted with a base oil.

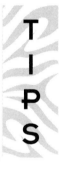

T
I
P
S

> *An effective lock moisturizer is a light rose water and glycerine spray.*

The following list contains carrier or base oils used to mix with other essential oils. Base oils are generally fruit, vegetable, or plant oils.

Base Oils

Sweet almond—Soothing to the skin; contains minerals and vitamins and is rich in protein. It relieves dryness, reduces itching, and reduces inflammation.

Apricot—Contains minerals and vitamins. Apricot is good for all hair and skin types and is an excellent emollient to soften dry hair.

Avocado—Enriched with vitamins, protein, and lecithin (which is an antioxidant), avocado is an excellent emollient and natural emulsifier. Avocado is great on all skin types. It is an effective remedy for eczema and it absorbs well into the skin.

Borage seed—High in amino acid (linolenic), vitamins, and minerals. It has excellent rejuvenating and stimulating properties.

Coconut—An emollient for all hair types; coconut softens hair.

Jojoba—A waxy substance, similar to natural sebum, that replaces collagen. Jojoba has high penetration to hair and scalp and controls flaking.

Olive oil—Absorbs well, is soothing to the scalp, and contains vitamins and minerals.

Peanut oil—Contains protein, amino acids. Peanut oil is good for all hair types.

Safflower oil—It is high in lecithin and is a good base for non-mixing substances. It contains amino acids, protein, minerals, and vitamins.

Sesame oil—It contains lecithin, amino acids, protein, minerals, and vitamins. Sesame oil fights psoriasis and eczema.

Soy bean—It contains proteins, minerals, and vitamins. Soy bean can be used on all hair types.

Sunflower oil—It contains vitamins and minerals. Sunflower oil can be used on all hair types.

Shea butter—It is an excellent emollient, prevents dryness, regenerates skin cells, helps healing and absorbs into hair and scalp. Shea butter strengthens hair by re-moisturizing.

Castor oil—It has excellent absorption properties, is soothing and lubricating to the skin. Castor oil contains hydroxy acid.

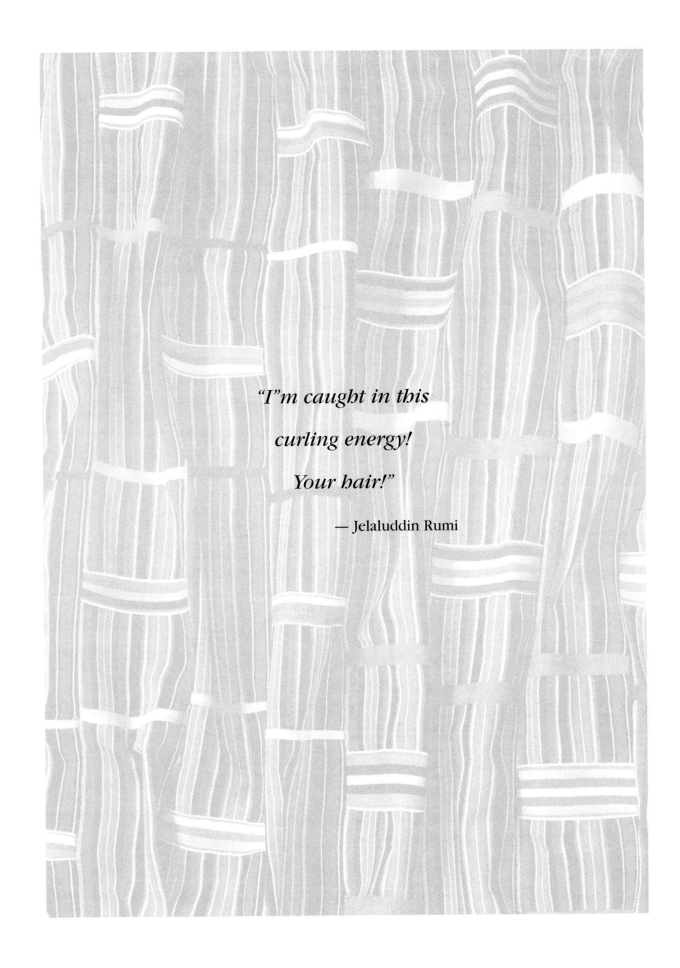

"I"m caught in this

curling energy!

Your hair!"

— Jelaluddin Rumi

CHAPTER

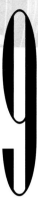

Textured Hair is Manageable

KNOWLEDGE BOX

In this chapter you will learn:

1

To identify hair crafters' tools and how to
handle them to create braiding styles

2

How to brush and comb out textured hair safely

3

How to section hair to prepare for various braiding designs

4

Shampoo and massaging techniques

5

How to apply and use various hair oils
and conditioning preparations

INTRODUCTION

Natural hair is virgin hair, not altered by chemical or thermal services. Natural hair care, in turn, is the process by which the hair service enhances that natural state.

It is a holistic approach to hair care. This approach recognizes the integrated balance between the body, mind, and spirit. The services provided are generally gentle, wholesome, corrective, and nurturing to the entire body.

Environmentally safe products or non-toxic products are often a part of the service. Products made of plants, fruits, vegetables, herbs, or essential oils are often used during these therapeutic services.

Most importantly, natural hair care preserves the original state of textured hair and makes it manageable through shampooing, grooming, braiding, extending, wrapping, twisting, weaving, cutting, and setting.

Products made of plants, fruits, vegetables, herbs, or essential oils are often used during therapeutic services.

A new approach to hair care is Natural Hair Care:
- *all textures are good or beautiful*
- *embellish the texture, don't alter it*

WHAT IS GROOMING?

The proper grooming of textured hair is a *nurturing* experience. Regular hair care and grooming will *encourage* new growth, *nourish* weakened or damaged hair, and *enhance* the overall aesthetics of hair.

Often, a client comes to the natural hair care specialist looking for nurturing rather than trying to obtain a trendy new hairstyle. Many are interested in braiding styles as a chemical-free approach to hair care. The specialist, through various braiding techniques and styles, is in a unique position to not only correct hair problems, but to promote the cultural aesthetics of natural hair without altering its texture through chemicals.

As a natural hair care specialist, your touch must be therapeutic. You will use more gentle massaging techniques when shampooing or rinsing. Your products are natural, aromatic, and soothing—not caustic. And, your approach to serving the client is one that brings together the emotional and physical health of the client.

For African-American clients in particular, the natural hair care specialist provides an essential service in helping both men and women embrace their distinctive hair. In this society, too many African-Americans are convinced that they do not possess natural beauty. However, one of our most distinguishing qualities is the differences in our hair textures—from kinky to soft waves. The astute stylist can redefine what is ethnically beautiful or "acceptable." And, by educating the client on how to take better care of their hair, the natural hair care specialist is an important catalyst in helping clients develop a healthier approach to self-image and self-acceptance.

The natural hair care specialist is important in helping clients develop a healthier approach to self-image.

Depending on whether the specialist is a barber, hair braider, or locktician, the term **grooming** can refer to different techniques and services. The person that specializes in locking techniques is often referred to as a locktician. A locktician only grooms locks, and is generally well versed in herbal rinses and natural hair conditioners that embellish and strengthen the hair.

Locked hair is groomed differently than hair that is being prepared for braiding, weaving, or cutting. A locktician, as do most hair braiders, refers to grooming as "cultivating" the hair for style development and nurturing and finishing natural hair to enhance the overall beauty of the style. The proper maintenance and grooming of locked hair will be discussed in chapter 10.

To groom the hair is to comb, brush, or style in its natural textured state. Whether it is before a technique or during the styling process, grooming is where the *nurturing* and the *healing* process begin.

Also, a stylist must be able to identify the variety of coil patterns in textured hair in order to safely groom and prevent breakage. Once these patterns are identified—through professional consultation, client information, observation, shampoo, and rinse preparations—the stylist must then choose the proper tools.

TOOLS OF THE CRAFT

A braid stylist is an artist, and like any other artist, the stylist creates the art with implements that are necessary to execute the finished product. The tools the stylist chooses are as essential to this profession as in any other craft. To complete a beautiful, lasting, natural braided look, you should use only the best and proper tools to assist in the service. (Fig 9.1)

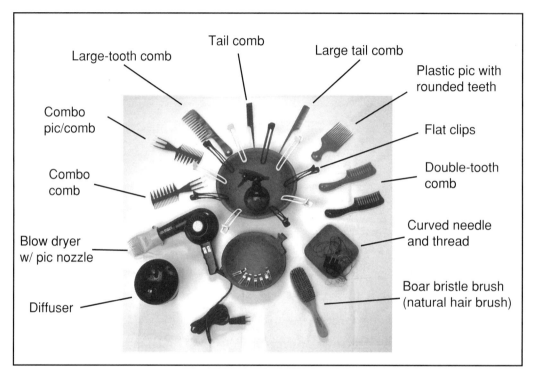

Figure 9.1 Tools of the craft

A list of your tools of the trade should include the following:

1. *Blow dryer with pic nozzle—Loosens the wave pattern in textured hair for braiding and weave styles. It dries, elongates, and softens textured hair. Use hard plastic pic nozzles (metal attachments become too hot).*

2. *Diffuser—Dries hair without disturbing the finished look, and avoids the use of direct heat which removes moisture.*

3. *Finishing comb—Usually 8 to 10 inches in length, great on fine or straight hair, and used while cutting hair.*

4. *Large-tooth comb—There are a large variety of shapes and designs available. The teeth of large-tooth combs should have long rounded tips to avoid scratching the scalp. In widths, the teeth can range from medium to large. The distance between the teeth, however, is the most important feature of this comb. Larger spacing will allow curly, kinky hair to move between the rows of teeth with ease. Large-tooth combs ply through hair with less snarling than smaller combs.*

5. *Tail comb—Ideal for parting hair to prepare for braiding styles. It is excellent for design parting and weaving, is easy to use for sectioning large segments of hair, and is excellent for aiding the opening and removal of braids.*

6. *Plastic pic with rounded teeth—Used for lifting and separating textured and curly hair such as Afros and human hair extensions. Teeth are long and spaced wide apart. They can be made of metal, plastic, wood, or ivory. Great for separating and lifting textured hair.*

7. *Double-tooth comb—Excellent on wet, curly hair, it is designed to limit tangling and snarling.*

8. *Curved needle—For weaving thread and used for braid weave styles and weaves. Curved needles are excellent for getting close to the scalp without sticking into the client's scalp.*

9. *Boar bristle brush (natural hair brush)—Best used to stimulate the scalp as well as a good tool to remove dirt and lint from locks. (Nylon bristled brushes are not as durable and many of them snag hair. Soft nylon brushes can be an option for fine, soft hair around the hairline.)*

10. *Spray bottle container—For use to comb out and finish a look, and to keep detangling solutions.*

11. *Long clips—To separate hair in large sections.*

12. *Butterfly and small clips—To separate hair in small and large sections.*

13. *Cutting comb—For cutting small sections. It should be used only after hair is softened and elongated with blow dryer.*

14. *Hands—Take care of them!*

15 *Mannequin—To practice styles and braid technique.*

16. *Vent brush—A wide-bristle plastic brush to be used on wet, wavy or curly, dry hair. It is excellent on human hair extensions. Vent brushes may have a single or a double row of*

teeth. Though it helps to detangle hair, the stylist must work gently so as not to snarl or snag kinky hair on teeth.

17. *Five-inch scissors—Necessary for finished look and to trim fringes and excess extension material. Used to create shape.*

18. *Hackle—A board of fine, upright nails that human hair gets combed through to detangle or blend colors and highlights.*

19. *Drawing board—Used to control human hair while braiding. Flat leather pads with very close and fine teeth that sandwich the human hair. The sandwich is weighed down to secure and is pulled in the required proportion without losing and disturbing the rest of the hair.*

20. *Hood dryer—Use this type of hair dryer to remove excess moisture before hand blow drying hair. The hood dryer eliminates excessive use of hand blow drying and reduces direct heat on the hair.*

21. *Other accessories—Butterfly clips, elongated and short metal clips, towels, and capes.*

N O T E S

Textured hair requires different tools than relaxed or straightened hair. Any implement that creates discomfort, snags, or pulls out hair must be discarded. All tools, including clips, should be easy to use and must be sanitized.

COMBING AND SECTIONING

Contrary to what many people may believe about kinky hair being tough, this textured hair (as natural hair care specialists prefer to call it) is very fragile when wet.

It is more elastic when dry. However, the normal exercise of stretching wet, textured hair can severely damage the hair shaft. The way most textured hair is structured—in a coil pattern—at each bend in the coil the hair strand is thinner, so there are several potential breakage points in each strand. As a matter of precaution, combing wet, textured hair should be very meticulous work. Remember: The more coil in the hair, the more fragile it is when wet. Stretching and pulling on these wet and fragile strands in order to detangle and prepare the hair is tedious, but it can be mastered.

Detangling Wet, Textured Hair

Detangling wet, textured hair can be made much easier by following an eight-step procedure:

1. *Start at the nape of the neck. Using a tail comb with large rounded teeth, divide the crown of the head in half from ear to ear. Use butterfly clips to separate, pinning away the front section from the back section.*

2. *Part the back of the head into four to six sections. For thick textured hair, make more sections to allow for ease and control. For thinner hair, use fewer sections. The front half of the head can be sectioned in three sections or more because the hair is less dense in the front. Separate sections with clips. Gently spray each section as you go along with a solution of 4 parts water with 1 part cream rinse or oil.*

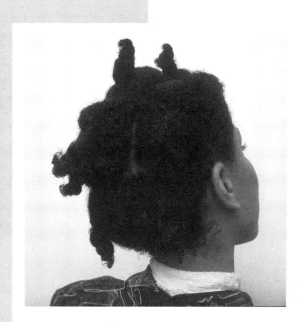

Figure 9.2 Hair sectioned

3. *Begin on the left section. There should be enough hair to hold in the palm of the hand. Too much hair in this section can cause you to lose control, which could result in hair breakage.*

4. *Holding the palm upward and close to the scalp, start combing with a large-tooth comb at the ends of the hair first, working your way up to the base of the scalp. Work from the bottom up because hair tangles at the ends.*

5. *The combing movement should be fast and rhythmic, but not so much as to put tension on the scalp. It is better to use a picking motion to comb through the hair.*

6. *Once the hair is combed thoroughly, the section can be divided into two equal parts and twisted together to the end, separating and holding the combed section in place. (Fig 9.2)*

7. *Repeat the above process for the other sections of the hair to finish the complete head.*

8. *Place the client under a medium heat hood dryer for approximately five minutes to remove excess water.*

TIPS

🌀 *When choosing your tools, rub your combs on the back of your hand. If they are scratchy, they are likely to irritate the client's scalp.*

🌀 *Spray with moisturizing/detangling solution as often as needed for detangling and softening. Very porous hair may absorb the water quickly.*

🌀 *With very coiled or kinky hair, a springing effect will be noticed in the combed section of the hair, as compared to the uncombed sections. You know then that the curl has been stretched and separated.*

BLOW DRYING TEXTURED HAIR

Why blow dry textured hair? Not only does it dry the hair quickly, it also softens the hair, making it manageable for easy combing. It loosens the wave patterns in the hair while stretching the shaft length. This is excellent for short hair, allowing for more long braiding styles.

1. *After the hair has been shampooed and properly sectioned, place the client under the hood dryer for five to ten minutes (depending on the density of the hair) to remove excess water.*

2. *Blow drying creams and lotions protect the hair from direct heat and help control the manageability of textured hair. These creams or lotions can be applied before each section, if combed thoroughly, and afterward.*

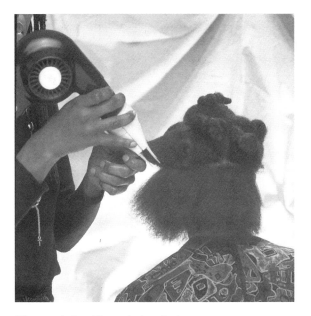

Figure 9.3   Blow drying hair.

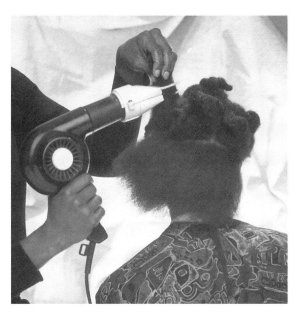

Figure 9.4   Blow drying hair.

There are several blow drying aids or conditioners that will coat the hair and protect it from excessive heat. All will allow the comb to glide with ease. Some have moisturizers in them, which can leave the hair feeling heavy and greasy. Instead, blow drying creams should be light and aromatic. They should have an oil or glycerine base without a greasy, tacky feel to the hand.

N
O
T
E
S

3. *Opening one of the combed sections, use a pic nozzle attachment on the blow dryer and begin drying using the comb-out motion.*

4. *Holding the hair down and away from the client's head, start the comb-out motion with the pic nozzle always pointing away from the client. As the end stretches, work the blow dryer, heat blowing downward, toward the scalp. Blowing directly into the scalp could burn. (Figs 9.3 and 9.4)*

5. *As the longer hair dries, some shorter lengths of hair may have curled closer to the scalp. In order to get closer to the scalp, reduce the heat and speed of the blow dryer. This allows the pic nozzle to reach shorter, more resistant textured hair and loosen the curl pattern.*

6. *After each section is dried, the hair is ready to be braided or styled.*

You should be aware that most clients receiving your services will have a history of chemically treated hair. While in transition to going "totally natural" or "in-between perms," the hair follicles are under an extreme amount of stress. Each strand has two textures: natural and chemical. At the point at which these two textures meet, the shafts are weak and may snap off in the comb-out and sectioning process. Be very gentle with hair in transition. In most cases, the client has experienced some form of hair damage or scalp irritation.

T I P S

🌀 *To minimize breakage and allow for easier blow drying, always use pre-conditioners or cream rinses, or natural oils and water to comb out hair.*

🌀 *When blow drying, use moderate heat.*

🌀 *Place client under hood dryer first to avoid excessive use of hand blow drying.*

🌀 *Remember that blow drying will stretch the hair. Avoid placing extreme heat on chemically treated hair that is already stressed. Concentrate on drying, not stretching, the hair. The two hair textures will never look the same unless you place extreme heat on the untreated hair.*

🌀 *What is extreme heat? If it is too hot for your hand when placed in front of the nozzle, it is too hot for the hair.*

PREPARING THE HAIR FOR BRAIDING

Preparing the hair for braiding means that the hair and scalp have been thoroughly cleaned. Hair should be dry, softened, and free of snarls.

1. *When you begin, look for bald, thinning, or damaged hair areas. These problem areas will determine the style of the braiding design. Texture, length, and hair condition will determine the style design around the problem areas.*

2. *Before you proceed with any braiding service, examine the scalp for scratches, abrasions, sores, irritations, birthmarks, or moles.*

3. *The crown is your canvas. Be certain that the natural hair and the client's scalp condition can support the braiding style that you chose.*

Hair Oil Preparation

Preparing the scalp for braiding also involves selecting a natural hair care product that will help soften the hair as well as moisten the scalp. The preparation should provide a light coat of moisture to the strands that will aid the braiding process. Natural hair oils have been part of the hair grooming process since the ancient Khamits.

The body, however, produces its own natural oil in the scalp called sebum. Sebum is produced by the sebaceous glands that are connected to the hair follicle. Sebum travels along the outside of the hair shaft, acting as a lubricant and natural emollient that seals in moisture. However, with textured hair, the spiral structure of the hair shaft makes it difficult for the sebum to travel along the shaft. In many cases, the scalp may be oily, but the hair remains dry because the sebum can not travel around the tightly coiled hair shaft.

The cellular structure of textured hair is different than other hair types. In the spiral pattern, the outer shingled layers of cells that protect the hair cuticle lie closer together, making the hair look drier than other hair types. The hair can become fragile in cases where the scalp has fewer sebaceous glands and produces less oil or sebum.

To replace the sebum, natural oils from plants and flowers can restore moisture and protect the hair. These oils add a thin lubricant for braiding, making both the client's natural hair and extension (if one is used) more pliable and softer on the braider's fingertips.

Heavy synthetic oils such as lanolin, petroleum, and mineral oils should be avoided because of their ability to attract dust and dirt. Olive oil, though not synthetic, is no substitute. It is far too heavy to groom the scalp, but can be used for hot oil treatments (see Chapter 8). Synthetic oils do not absorb into the scalp and often leave a coat of residue, which ultimately creates blockage at the follicle base. This will eventually hinder the growth process.

Hair can become fragile in cases where the scalp has fewer sebaceous glands and produces less oil or sebum.

Most hair oils are in liquid form. They should be light to the touch and absorbed quickly into the skin, leaving a light, soft sheen to the hair.

Pomades are scented hair oils that have a cream or wax base. Be careful when using pomades with heavy wax bases. When selecting pomades, a stylist should look for natural ingredients that will stimulate hair growth and lubricate. Pomades should not be greasy, sticky, or pasty. Heavy pomades will block pores and cause waxy build-up in the braids. Clots of wax build-up at the base of the braid are a major problem when removing braided styles. Wax from the heavy grease or pomade that is left in the hair collects dust and dirt from the environment. It then can become impacted or hardened between the new growth and hair extension. When combing out this wax residue, be careful to avoid breakage.

🐾 *Pull clumped residue apart by hand, using your fingers to loosen the wax.*

🐾 *Further removal requires the use of a large-tooth comb.*

🐾 *Lightly spray affected area with a water and cream rinse solution to soften build-up.*

🐾 *Always start at the ends of the hair, holding at the base so that the client is completely comfortable and hair is not overly stressed.*

**T
I
P
S**

"The world is a mirror:

show yourself in it and it

will reflect your image."

—African Proverb

C H A P T E R

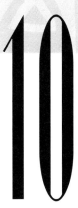

Braiding and Sculpting Techniques

K N O W L E D G E   B O X :

In this chapter you will learn:

1

Cornrowing (with and without extensions) techniques

2

Single braids (with and without extensions) techniques

3

Basic lock methods

4

An overview of texture and braid styles

INTRODUCTION

The following descriptions will provide you with the basic knowledge of the popular natural braid styles and techniques. The creative art form is unlimited, and the techniques offered here are fundamental and can be improvised to allow self expression. As demand increases for the natural braided look, the more diverse styles will become.

But more importantly, the stylist must be aware of the differences and options that are available to the client. It is through the complete understanding of naturally textured hair, the variety of braid styles, and above all the required hands-on experience and practice that will enable you to be among the best.

NATURAL STYLISTS AND BRAIDING TERMS

As the braid industry becomes more popular, innovative braid stylists will create more beautiful styling options. The names may vary from state to state; however, it is necessary to highlight the featured styles.

The following is a general description of the beginning level techniques:

🖉 *African Kurl (Twist Out)*

This style is achieved by using a double twist technique. The twisting technique is done wet in order to promote textures and waves. "Twist out" is the unravelling of the twist, adding fullness and a crimped effect.

🖉 *Afro*

This style can be achieved on long or short curly, kinky or wavy hair. Hair that is cut and textured can vary in its final shape.

🖉 *Afro Weave*

*This style is achieved by attaching textured hair on a **weft** to a designed cornrow basis. It is sewn with a cotton thread.*

🖉 *Braids (single or individual braids)*

These names are interchangeable for most braid stylists across the country. These techniques are basic "free hanging" braids with or without extensions. The braid is divided into three equal sections that are intertwined or weaved into one another.

Casama Braids

Large, single braids with a tight stitch; they are tapered and/or curved at the ends.

Cornrows and Canerows

Underhand three-strand braids, interwoven to lay flat on the scalp. They can be designed and sculpted into varying patterns with or without extensions.

Flat Twist

Two-sectioned braid, interwoven to lay flat on the scalp. It can be designed into varying patterns with or without extensions.

Geni-Locs

This style uses the single braid technique and wrapping technique. Yarn is used on this two-step procedure. Yarn gives a matte finish to resemble locks.

Goddess Braids

A large inverted braid designed to lay flat on the scalp in varying design patterns. The free end is styled into an updo finished style.

Locks, Dread Locks

Natural textured hair is intertwined and meshed together to form a single or separate network of hair.

Nu-locs

This technique is done with yarn fiber giving the extension a matte finish like locks. A single braid based technique is used.

Nubian Coils

This technique is styled on naturally curly or textured hair. Hair is curled into a cylindrical shape with a comb or hands.

Lin Twist

This technique resembles the flat twist and is performed with lin fiber.

Silky Twist

Large sections like a cornrow base are rolled and gelled into a flat design pattern.

Silky Wrap or Silky Loc

This style is a two-step process. First, the braid extension is applied; then the synthetic hair is wrapped around the braid. (Fig 10.1)

CORNROWS

There are many techniques to starting the traditional on-the-base braid known as the cornrow. The cornrow is created with a three-strand, on-the-scalp braid which uses an underhand "pick-up" technique. The fundamental of braiding starts with the basic cornrow. According to master braid designer Annu Prestonia, co-owner of Khamit Kinks in New York and Georgia and celebrity braid designer (among her clients are such notables as Stevie Wonder and Angela Basset) cornrows are the foundation of all braid styles. "If you excel at the art of cornrowing, all other braiding techniques are at your disposal," says Prestonia.

To cornrow like a professional you must be patient and practice. A skilled braider must take the time daily to practice cornrowing. Cornrowing is the repetition of the entire woven patterns; the sequence of weave patterns may vary and will determine the style. However, the series of revolutions are a simple repetitive motion of secure pick-up motion. Practicing on a mannequin will help to develop speed, accuracy and finger/wrist dexterity. Braid services can vary in time from two hours for a large braid to two days for a micro braid. Mastering the basic cornrow technique will enable you to approach other braid styles with confidence.

Skillful cornrowing is designed through the process of sculpting the parted sections. Sculpting is more than just vertical or horizontal partings. When sculpting the braid, you must first visualize the finished look. This will allow you to create smooth and consistent curved partings that contour with the head. The curve partings are a part of the design, so they must be neat and even. The more creative you are in designing the parts, the more beautiful the finished sculpted look will be. This contouring or sculpting is especially beautiful on small to medium sized cornrows.

Three-Strand Cornrow

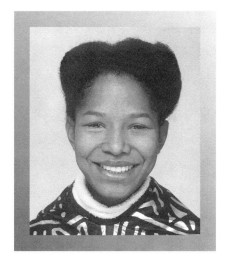

Before

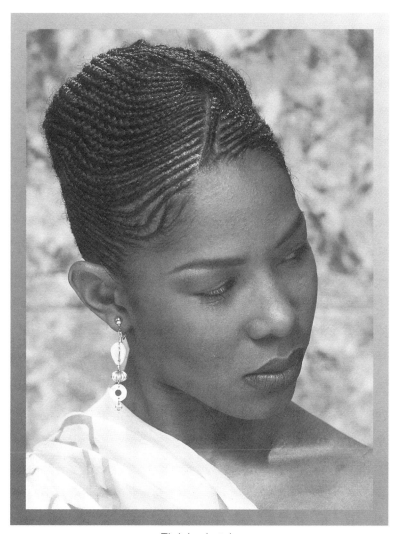

Finished style

Practice the following technique for cornrowing. It uses three strands with an underhand weaving motion, in which the strands on the sides are always passed under the center strand, alternating from the right side to the left, and left side to the right. Tulani Kinard, master braider and owner of Tulani's Regal Movement in New York, gives the following technique:

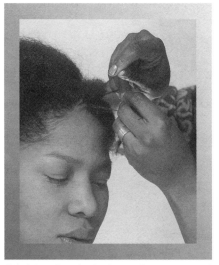

Divide the hair into three equal parts.

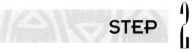

STEP 1

Begin by taking a section as small as you want the braid to be. Divide the section into three equal strands. Start at the hair line (depending on the style, the braid can begin anywhere from the nape of the neck forward). The strand on the far left will be called strand 1, the center is strand 2, and the strand on the far right is strand 3.

STEP 2

Cross the left strand 1 under center strand 2. Center strand 2 is now on the left and strand 1 is the new center. Passing the strand under the center with each revolution creates the underhand cornrow braid.

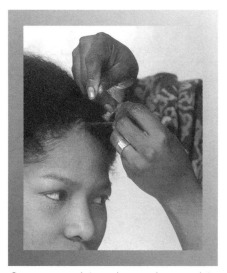

Cross strand 1 underneath strand 2.

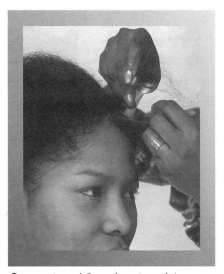

Cross strand 3 under strand 1.

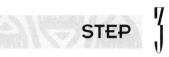

STEP 3

With each crossing under, or revolution, you must pick up new equal size sections of hair and add them to the center strand 2; pick up before crossing the outer strands under the center strand. Now cross strand 3 under strand 1. At the end of this revolution, strand 3 is the new center.

STEP 4

Each time you make a revolution (crossing under the center strand), you must pick up the hair from the scalp and add it to the new center. With each revolution, alternate the side of the braid on which you pick up hair.

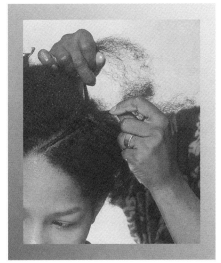

Pass strand 2 under strand 3. Work from side to side.

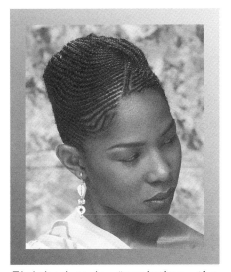

Finished style, "sculpting—the three-strand cornrow"

STEP 5

As you move along the section, cornrowing and picking up more hair, you add fullness to the braid. The braids appear to be closer together. Contoured parting should be clean and neat.

Cornrows with Extension

Hair additions or extensions are used for the following reasons:

- *to lengthen short hair*
- *to add volume to thin hair*
- *to protect damaged hair*
- *to add dimension to the height of the natural hair*
- *to allow the braid style to last longer*
- *to make a creative and cultural statement*

Cornrow with Extension (Feed-in method)

The feed-in method can be applied to cornrows or individual braids. There are several different methods for integrating extension hair into the hairline. Some methods just introduce large amounts of extension material to the fragile hairline, leaving the front of the braid bulky and knotted. In some cases, this bulky, bumpy look has become very popular. It is a fast and effective method for adding extensions if the client does not mind the braids looking like a helmet!

But many braid professionals contend that the braid extension should be concealed and the knot or lump eliminated because it is damaging to the hair. "When hair is braided using the knot or lump at the beginning of the braid, it is a tell-tale sign that you are wearing an extension," notes Taliah Waajid, author of *Hairitage Masterpieces*. She uses the feed-in method to gradually add hair throughout the braid. Literally, strand by strand the braid must be built up. Too large amounts of extension material places excessive weight on the fragile areas of the hairline. It also tightens and pulls the hair and creates an unrealistic finished look. By properly applying the correct tension application with the feed-in method, the braid stylist can eliminate the artificial look.

The traditional cornrow does not look like a hat of braids. It is flat, natural, and contoured to the scalp. The parting is definitely important because it defines the finished style. The feed-in method creates a tapered or narrow base at the hairline. As small pieces or strips of extension hair are added, the base fills in, bringing the adjoining braids closer together.

This technique takes longer to perform. However, the cornrow lasts longer, looks more natural, and does not put excessive tension on the hairline. Practice this method for a flat contour, natural cornrow style.

The Feed-in Method

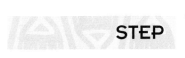 **STEP** 1

Start at the hairline by parting off a corn-row base in the desired style.

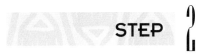 **STEP** 2

At the starting point, no extension added. If the hair extension is required because of a thinning hairline, minute amounts can be applied five to ten strands. This is all relative to the size of the cornrow.

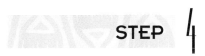 **STEP** 3

Divide the natural hair into three equal portions.

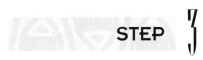 **STEP** 4

With the first revolution, left strand 1 crosses **under** strand 2.

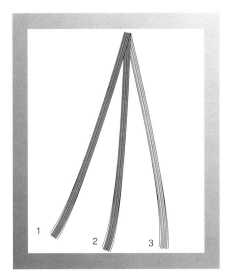

Three-strand extension

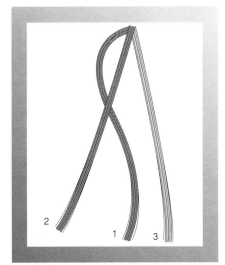

First revolution

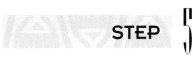 **STEP** 5

On the second revolution, the right strand 3 crosses **under** strand 1. A small portion of natural hair is picked up and added to the outside portion during the revolution.

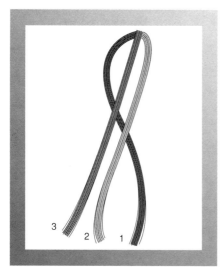

Second revolution

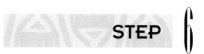

STEP 6

On the third revolution, bring strand 3 to the center strand, picking up a small portion at the base of natural hair.

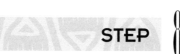

STEP 7

After several revolutions and pick ups, apply small amounts of folded extensions under the natural hair, to the center and ouotside portions. Hair extension must be tucked into the fold of the two adjoining portions.95 The amount of extension should be proportionately less than the size of the base.

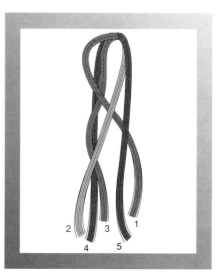

Third revolution

STEP 8

The folded extension is always applied to the center and outside portions before the pick up. Do not forget to pick up natural hair with **each** revolution to execute on the base cornrow.

NOTES

There are several different ways to start a cornrow and feed in extension pieces. Experiment with as many methods as you can. Different hairlines and styles require different methods.

Over-Directing Braid Extension

Precision parting and sectioning is vital to all braiding techniques. Parting will determine the direction of the braid. Clean and precise partings are required to create a strong braid base. Hair strands must never be over-directed or misplaced within an adjacent braid. If single strands are incorporated into another section outside of its own section, the hair will eventually break. Over-extending the hair adds tension to the unsupported strand.

During the cornrow process, when picking up hair at the base, the hair directly underneath the previous revolution must be incorporated into the braid. The hair picked up must never come from another subsection or be extended up into the braid from a lower part of the braid.

The same is true when applying any braid technique. When creating an individual braid with extensions, start in the center of the subsection. Over-extending or misplacing the beginning of the extension leaves the hair exposed and unsupported, which can led to breakage and traction alopecia. This is particularly true when adding extensions to the hairline. If the extension is not secure (2 or 3 revolutions before picking up), the extension will move away from the point of entry. This pulled base around the hairline will definitely create breakage and eventually alopecia.

For professional finishing, always trim or remove split ends that may pop through the braid shaft. Hold scissors flat, moving up the braid shaft. Avoid cutting into the braid.

T
I
P
S

Senegalese Twists

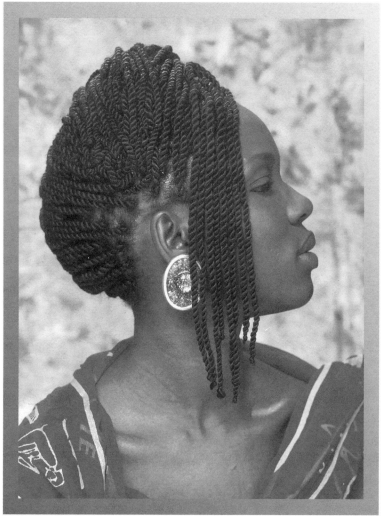
Finished style

Senegalese twists have their origin in West Africa. These braids are created using lin, synthetic material, kanekalon, or yarn extension material. It uses a two-strand braiding technique. Pre-plan the final style to determine how much material you will need. This will be determined by the length of the desired extension and the size of the partings. Separate and cut to the desired length.

Preparing hair and scalp

1. Shampoo; apply hot oil treatment; blow dry.

2. Match extension material to the client's hair color and texture.

STEP 1

Start by dividing the entire head in half from ear to ear.

STEP 2

Slightly above the ear with tail of comb, make a 45-degree part down toward the neck. The part can be as large or small as required for the size of the twist you are trying to create.

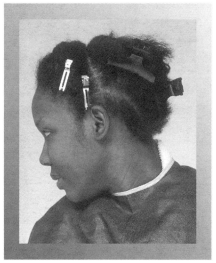

Part hair at 45-degree angle.

STEP 3

Make a subsection above the ear. Separate the subsection into two equal parts. Section off a required amount of extension material. Place the extension strip between the two equal parts.

STEP 4

Simultaneously, you must perform two twisting motions. The first twisting is to roll the fiber between both of your fingers, which secures the natural hair into the fiber. The second twisting motion takes the "rolled" fiber and hair, and twists or overlaps one strand over the other. This rolling motion is done with the finger tip and should be very tight.

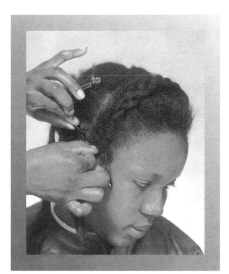

Roll fiber three or four times.

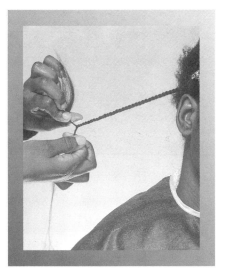

Twist one strand over the other to create a tight twist.

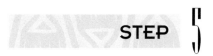
STEP 5

Continue the double twist motion for the entire length of the strand. Roll and cross strands until you reach the ends. Loop and knot the twists to close. Trim excess fiber.

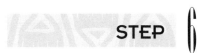
STEP 6

Seal ends with singeing method or knot and cut close.

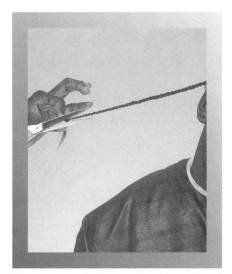

Seal the ends in the predetermined fashion.

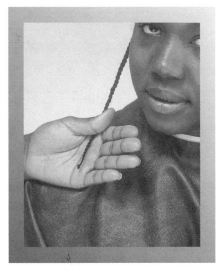

Finished sealed ends.

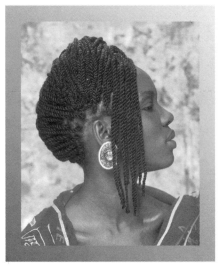

Finished style

Diamond Casama Braids

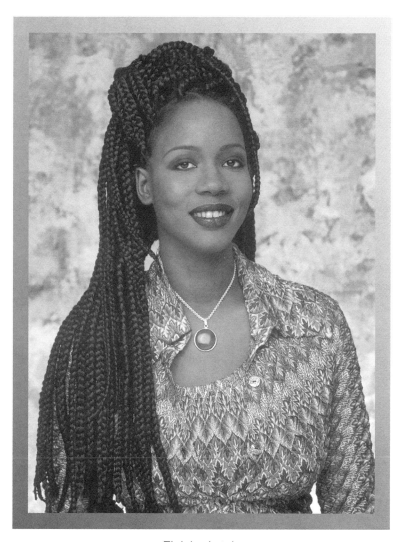

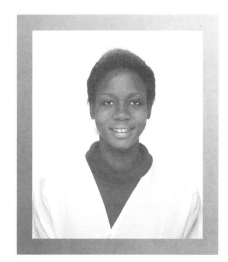

Before

Finished style

Casamas are created by using individual partings and braids that are larger in size than box braids or single braids. This technique requires three-strand braiding. The stitch of the braid itself is very tight, which allows the braid to curve when finished. The technique begins at the nape, where square, triangular, or rectangular partings are taken in any size desired. For the typical triangular style, triangles are one-half to one-inch. The first two or three rows from the nape up can be horizontal; when you reach the top, pre-plan your design based on whether an asymmetrical look is desired or not. If it is, create a side part and plan to create braids that begin at the part line and move across the top of the head. This means the partings will follow an angled line and will not be perfectly horizontal at the top.

When the entire head is completed in the desired fashion, the free-hanging braids are singed with a burner. Senior braid stylist Fanta Kaba of Tendrils, New York, performs this technique.

STEP 1

Start in the back of the head by parting a diagonal section at about a 45-degree angle, toward the front hairline, just past the ear. This section can be from 1 to 2" wide.

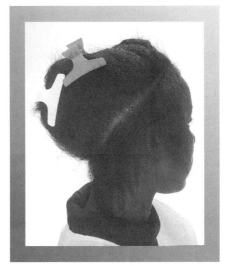

Parting hair at 45-degree angle.

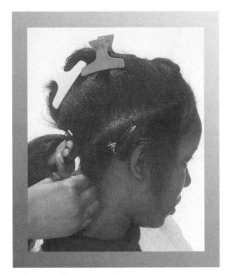

Diagonal sub-partings

STEP 2

Part the base into subsections with vertical parts to create the diamond sections. After subsection size has been determined, select the appropriate amount of Kanekalon. For tapered ends, the extension material is gently pulled at both sides so that the ends have a "shredded" uneven effect.

STEP 3

Take a strand of synthetic hair in a prede-termined length and fold it in half. Position the center of the strand at the base of the parting and wrap one half two or three revolutions around the base of the parted natural hair (base wrap is optional).

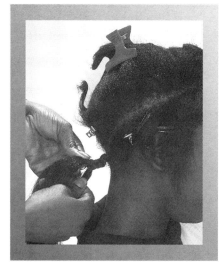

Three-strand braiding

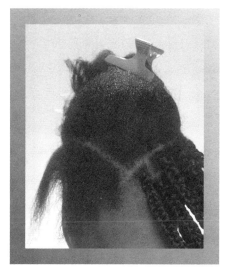

"V" shape partings

STEP 4

Immediately divide the hair into three sections, with the natural hair encom-passed into the center section. Make certain that the natural hair is concealed under the section before you begin three-strand braiding.

STEP 5

Alternate diagonal partings so that a "V" shape configuration is created in the back.

STEP 6

Partings should appear from front to back. Partings in front are curved and continue the diamond shape.

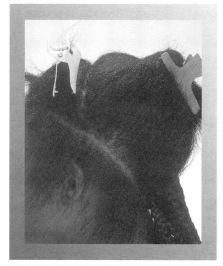

Front to back partings

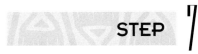 **STEP 7**

Braid the hair from scalp to ends, using an underhand or inverted technique. Each time you pass a side strand under the center strand, bring the center strand over tightly, so that the side strand becomes the new center strand. Then pass the alternate side strand under this one.

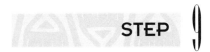 **STEP 8**

When you reach the ends, pull out a long, small section of hair, wrap it around the braid, knot it and repeat wrapping and knotting. This holds the tight braid in place and allows it to curve. Then continue to the next parting and repeat the entire procedure. Move up on the head, taking partings according to the pre-planned design.

STEP 9

When the entire head is completed, you can heat-seal the ends.

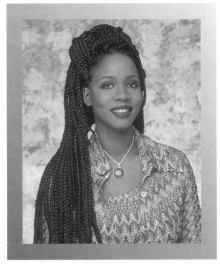

Finished style—diamond casama braids

Braid Tapering

The beauty of the casama braid is that the braid is full and wide at the base and tapered off at the ends. The tapered ends usually have a slight curve. To create this effect, the extension material must be shed before applying it to the head.

1. *Hold the required amount of extension material with two hands, about 6 to 10" apart.*

2. *Slowly pull the hair extension until it becomes uneven at the ends. By staggering at the ends, the extension material loses its blunt edges.*

3. *When staggering or redistributing extension material in an uneven matter, be aware of the length and size of the braid.*

Cornrows and Senegalese Twist (Combo)

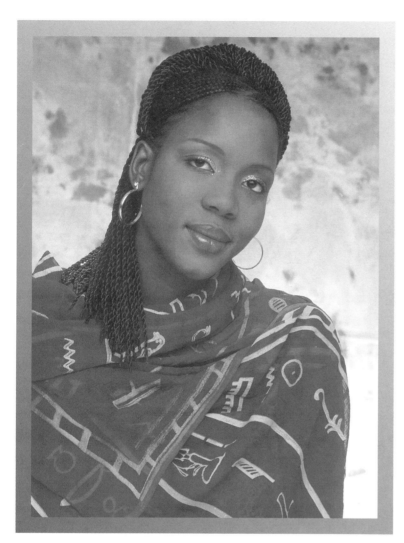

Finished style

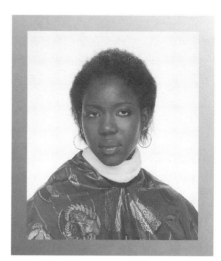

Before

This classic combination of micro cornrows and small Senegalese twists was sculpted by Avion Julien of Tulani's Regal Movement of New York.

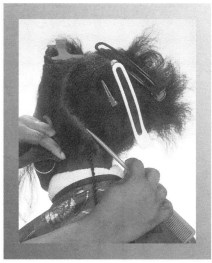

Senegalese twist back—45-degree angle

Part One

STEP 1

Start in the back by making a diagonal 45-degree angle section to just above the client's ear. Part off a subsection by making a smaller vertical part to the bottom of the neck.

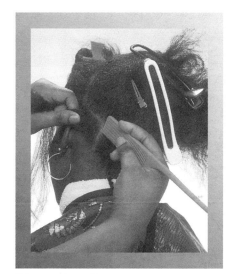

Diagonal parting

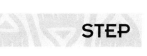**STEP 2**

Divide the subsection into two equal parts.

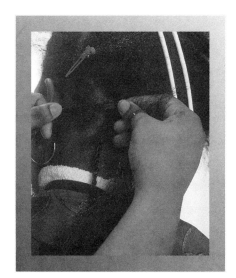

Two equal partings

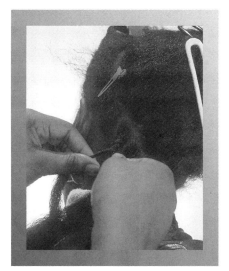

Hold and twist.

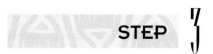

STEP 3

Double twist motion—roll hair strands counter-clockwise.

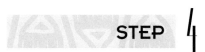

STEP 4

Once the extension is twisted close to the scalp, cross over the two twisted strands. The roll-overlap-roll sequence must be repeated for the entire twist. Tension must be consistent so that the twist remains straight.

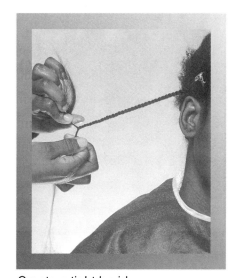

Create a tight braid.

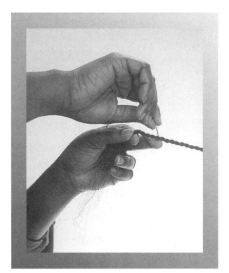

Loop to close.

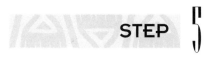

STEP 5

To close, loop ends by separating small numbers of strands and wrapping them around the braid. Singe ends secure and seal at the desired length.

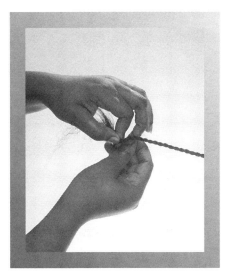

Complete loop.

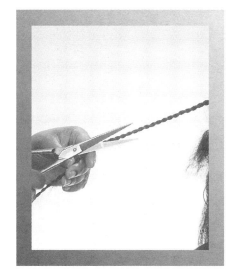

Trim.

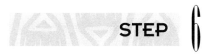 **STEP** 6

Trim frizzies or split ends from the twist to complete finished style.

Part Two

Cornrow Front with Extension

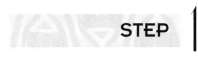 **STEP** 1

Start at the hairline by parting off the base in the desired size. Vertical parts should be about 1/4" wide.

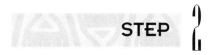 **STEP** 2

Divide the base into three equal portions. Take a pre-measured strip of extension proportionately less than the size of the base. Using the feed-in method, apply small units of extension (ten to twenty hairs) to the hairline.

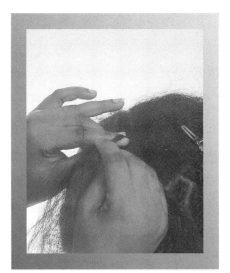

Pick up hair from the base and add to strand.

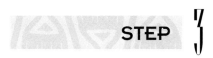

STEP 3

Begin the cornrow method. Each time you cross a strand from the outside to the inside center strand, pick up natural hair from the base and add it to the new center strand.

STEP 4

With your middle finger, hold the revolution in place. A second strip of extension can be added again to the left and outside strand.

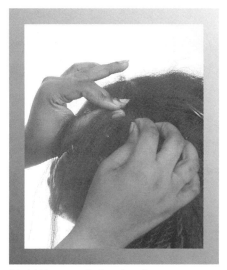

Hold the revolution in place.

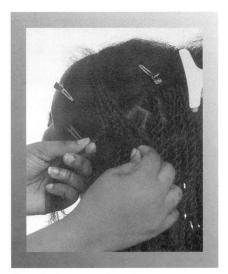

Create two equal portions.

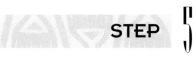

STEP 5

After the cornrow base is completed, start the Senegalese twist motion by separating the center strand and adding it to the outside pieces, creating two equal portions.

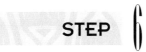 STEP 6

Continue by starting the double twist motion in order to create the Senegalese twist.

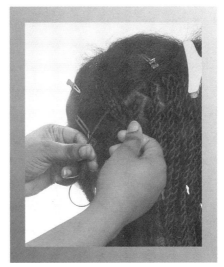

Roll and twist.

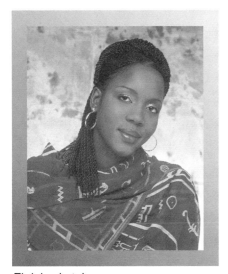

Finished style

STEP 7

Continue until you reach the end. Loop close, trim, and singe ends.

INDIVIDUAL BRAIDS

Individual braids may also be known as single or box braids. These are the most versatile to wear and they are directional—able to move or sweep into updos.

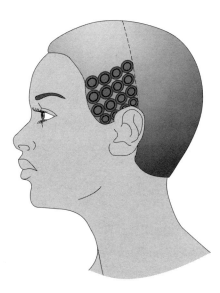

Twist or single braids placement

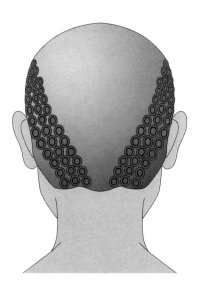

Twist or single braids placement—parting, sectioning, units

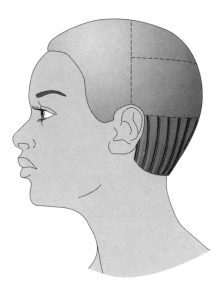

Cornrow—sectioning, parting

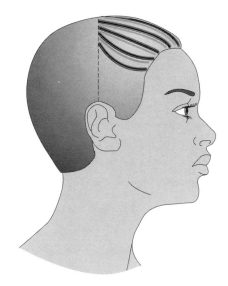

Cornrow placement—parting, sectioning

Whether the stylist uses human or synthetic extension or yarn, the variations of the braid are unlimited. Individual braids are traditional and classic. They are as fundamental as cornrows. Skill and practice are necessary in order to master this technique. The individual braid is a three strand braid that, if done improperly, can create excessive tension and lead to breakage.

The secrets to an excellent single braid are the following:

1. *The three portions are equal in size (uniform).*
2. *The braid is consistent and taut.*
3. *The braid is straight.*
4. *The base of the braid does not have a large loop or knot, putting excessive tension on the natural hair.*
5. *The braid must be tightly woven but done without pain to the client.*
6. *Parts should be consistent. As you get to the hairline braids should be parted to camouflage any thin areas. This can be done using angled or* **brick layered** *parts.*

T
I
P
S

Individual Braid

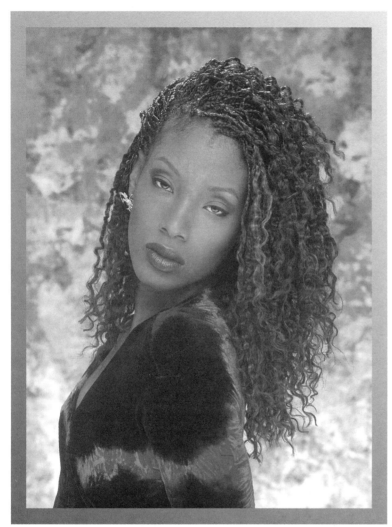

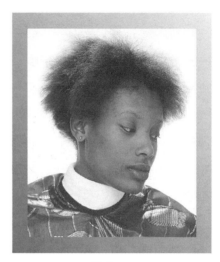

Before

Finished style (shown with Diva Crimp enhancement)

Braid stylist Susan Bishop of Jaha Studio in Silver Springs, MD, uses this technique for the individual braid style.

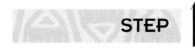

STEP 1

Part the hair in half from ear to ear.

Geni-Locs

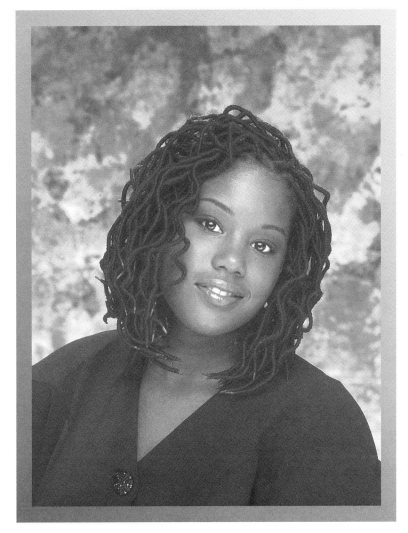

Finished style

Geni-Locs is a style that uses yarn as an extension. It is one of the hair locking alternatives that offers the client the benefit and beauty of locks without committing to locks permanently. They are versatile and can be bent and twisted into many different shapes to adorn the face. The Geni-Loc involves a braid-wrap technique to accomplish its finished look.

This technique is a specialty of braid designer Debra Hare-Bey of Red Creative Salon in New York.

STEP 1

Cut yarn at least twice the desired finished length. Give yourself enough length because the yarn must be folded before adding to natural hair.

STEP 2

Separate four pre-determined sizes of hair to start the first braid. Loop two pieces of yarn within the two pieces; then divide into three equal portions.

STEP 3

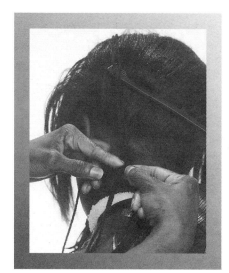

Pull out two pieces for wrap.

Begin the braid by placing looped pieces of extension on the three equal strands of natural hair. After the second revolution, pull out two pieces of yarn from the center for the wrapping. Continue to braid with the remaining pieces. Four pieces still remain, leaving one piece for the left strand 1, two pieces for the center strand 2, and one piece for the right strand 3.

STEP 4

Braid down the entire length.

STEP 5

Hold the braid close to the base with your left hand. Take two free pieces and begin to wind under and around the braid. With each revolution, move slightly down the braid so that the yarn does not overlap.

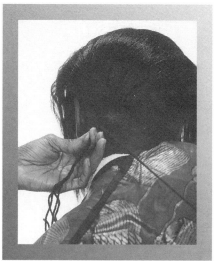

Wrap yarn under and around entire braid.

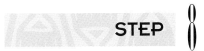 **STEP** 6

Continue the wrapping movement until the ends are reached. Braid ends closed. Trim the braid shaft to complete the braid style.

STEP 7

Singe braided ends and mold with fingers. Cut singed ends to remove excess material. Reburn if necessary to shape ends.

STEP 8

The front is parted on the diagonal for the design and to create fullness.

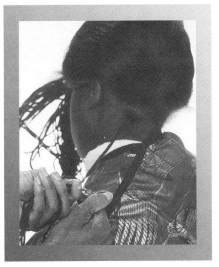

Single braid ends.

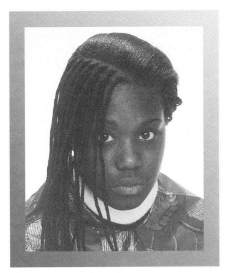

Front diagonal part

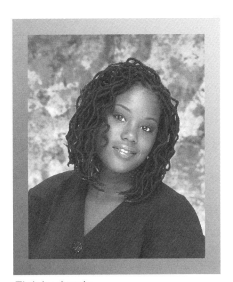

Finished style

THE AFRO WEAVE

Afros are back! They are fun, versatile, and can be extended to any color, length, or shape. The Afro weave adds a new dimension to textured hairstyling. This weave can be done with synthetic hair, human hair or yak, and human hair blends. The look is as contemporary today as it was in the 1960s. Weaving in hair can protect natural hair that has been chemically damaged. It covers balding or thinning spots, allowing the natural hair to grow.

The style that is featured in this section uses a yak and human hair blend. This blend offers a look that is close to natural. It is soft, yet the texture is very tight and coily. It is a customized blend that is sewn on a weft (hair sewn together to create a single line edge or strip.) The weft will be sewn on to a **track** (cornrows designed into a pattern for the foundation to place a weave extension).

N O T E S

When adding extensions, color and texture must match the client's own hair. When using a spiral synthetic hair for the finished look, separate each spiral curl for a fuller curly style.

The Afro "Congo Crown"

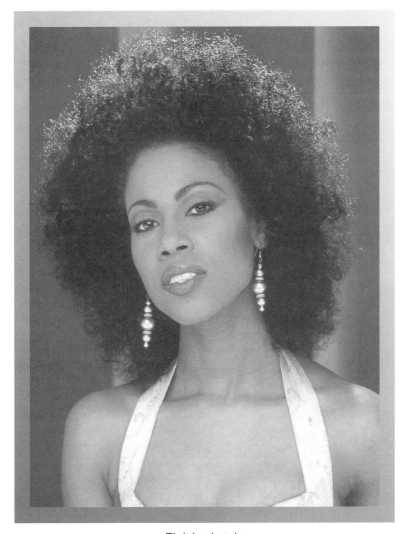

Finished style

STEP 1

Measure and separate 1 to 2" of the client's natural hairline around the entire head. Clamp away or braid down the hairline to separate it from the loose hair during the process. (You can do this with one large cornrow around the hairline.) Follow the natural hairline and begin the foundation for the weave by parting a small base in a circular pattern around the head to begin a small cornrow track.

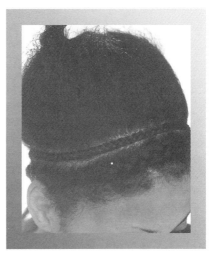

Parting small base—circular pattern

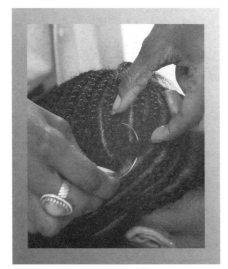

Zig-zag pattern

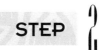

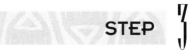

STEP 2

Cornrow in a circular pattern twice around the head. Keep cornrows flat and thin to avoid bulk. At the top of the crown, start a zig-zag pattern down the head. Keep within the circle. Extend cornrows past the length of the client's hair.

STEP 3

Once the foundation or track has been laid, take the excess braid which is not on the scalp, fold it on to the track at the crown of the head, and sew it or attach it.

STEP 4

With all the ends folded, sewn, and tucked away, the hair is ready for the wefted extension.

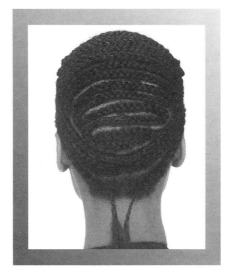

Fold and sew.

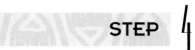

STEP 5

With a double loop "lock-in" stitch, attach the weft to the cornrowed track. Pull the needle through the weft and the bottom of the braid as you secure the track with your opposite hand. Pull the needle up until a small loop remains, then insert the needle twice through the loop and pull it tight.

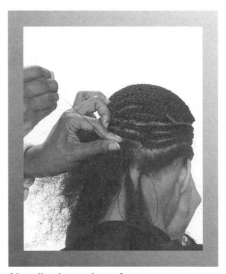

Needle through weft.

STEP 6

Follow the cornrow track around the head by positioning loops about 1/4" apart. Continue until the entire track is placed and secure the ends by inserting the needle through the loop three or four times.

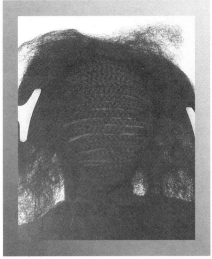

Track around head.

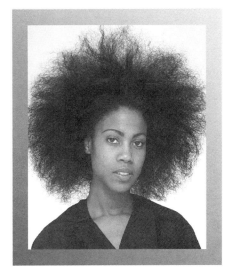

Secure track and complete.

STEP 7

Continue to sew and loop with the pre-measured track for the zig-zag section of the head.

STEP 8

Once the weave is secure, open up the loose cornow that you first made around the hairline. Then, incorporate the natural hair with the extension. Hair may be set on perm rods to add texture and curl.

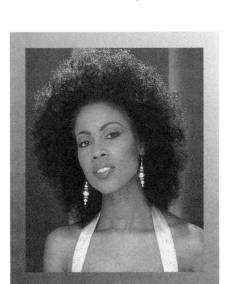

African weave "Congo Crown"— finished style

Pixie Braids

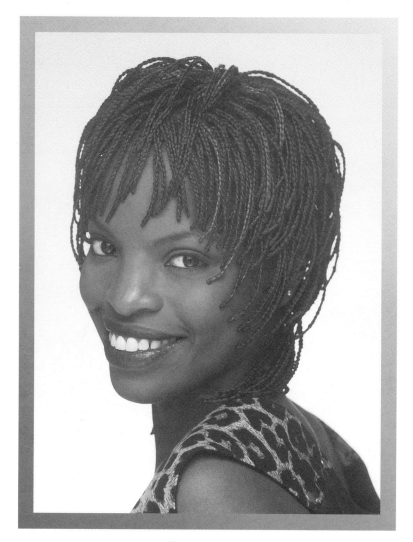

Finished style

The pixie braid style offers the client a youthful, short braid look. These individual braids are usually small to medium in size. The braids are layered to various lengths, usually framing the face. It is best to use a Kanekalon synthetic hair because this fiber singes better when molding the tips. The ends are cut and singed closed for the desired length.

The pixie braid must be tight. This will create a curved braid. There should be a light, airy feel to the braids. The layers create the feathered look by singeing the tips wherever necessary to complete the style. Always be aware of the client's natural hair length so that you do not burn their hair. The client's hair must be short for this technique and the finished braid can be slightly longer than the natural length. Singe the braid 1 to 2" longer than the client's natural hair.

STEP

Follow steps of individual braid instruction to start pixie braids.

STEP 2

Maintain the three-strand, outside-to-inside strand underhand braiding technique. Keep the braid stitch close.

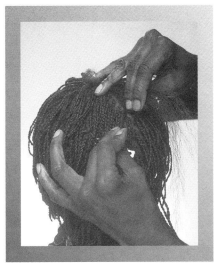

Three-strand braid sequence

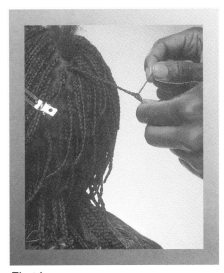

First loop

STEP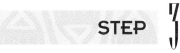

To hold the tight stitch taut, double loop the ends. Bring together the three strands; hold in one hand. With the other hand, separate several strands away from the braid, loop over and around, and pull through the loop. Repeat.

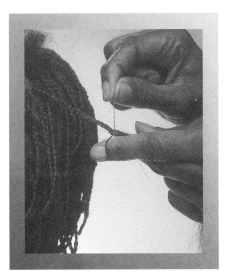

Second loop

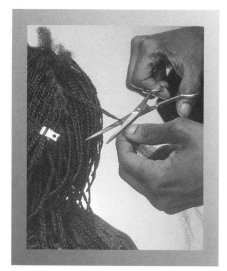

Trim.

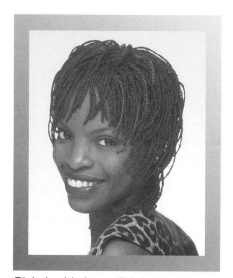

Pixie braid shag—finished style

STEP 4

Trim directly under the knot. Singe the knot to close. The singed ends will be warm and soft enough to mold by rolling the melted synthetic fiber between thumb and pointer finger. This will give the ends a sharp, pointed, neat finish.

Flat Twists

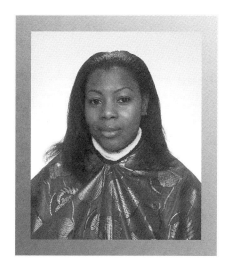

Before

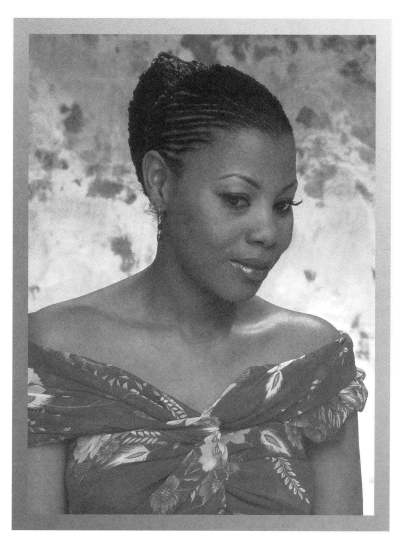

Finished style

Flat twists are a great alternative for clients with medium to shoulder-length hair. These twists are regal, soft, and easily sculpted into a day or evening look. Flat twists are a wonderful option for women interested in wearing their hair natural, but who do not want extensions or a woven braided look. Whether the hair is relaxed or chemical-free, this sculpted style offers an elegant and sophisticated crown of glory.

The flat twist is a two-strand, flat-on-the-scalp braid. The pattern resembles a flat spiral on a candy cane. Master braider Cecelia Hinds of Uzuri Braids in Washington, D.C. uses this technique. Two strands of equal proportions are twisted onto the scalp, picking up natural hair with every revolution. Most flat twist styles can last for two to three weeks.

To maintain this style, no shampooing is required. Cover nightly with a satin scarf. Oil scalp as needed.

"Lin Twist"—Flat Twist with Lin

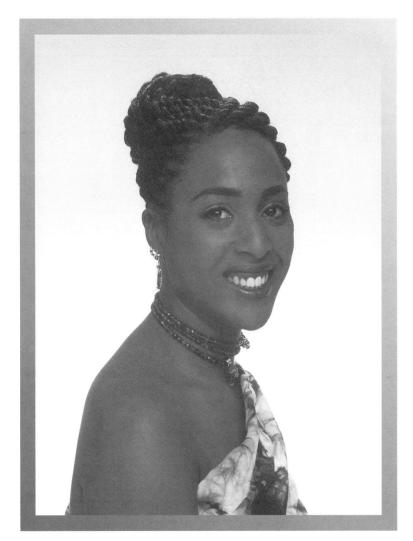

Finished style

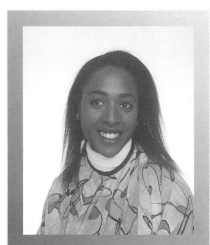

Before

Lin twists are the new classic to updo braiding styles. They give medium to shoulder-length hair dimension and diversity. The style can last three to four weeks. It can be done in two hours and is a quick alternative for clients who want extensions incorporated into their braid style. This technique also has been mastered by Cecelia Hinds of Uzuri Braids.

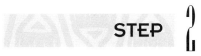 **STEP** 1

The two-strand twist can be performed by the roll-and-twist method at the hairline. Place the lin flat on top of the two equal portions. Secure the lin to each base with the double twist sequence, picking up natural hair with each revolution.

STEP 2

Pre-plan the style so that it contours with the client's head along the sides and back.

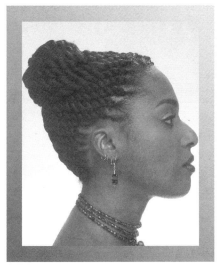

Lin twist—side

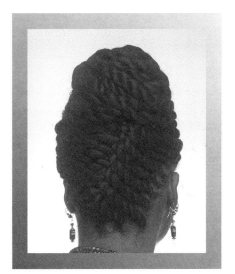

Lin twist—back

STEP 3

Gather the extended ends into a french roll or inverted cornrow; pin and tuck.

Silky Twist

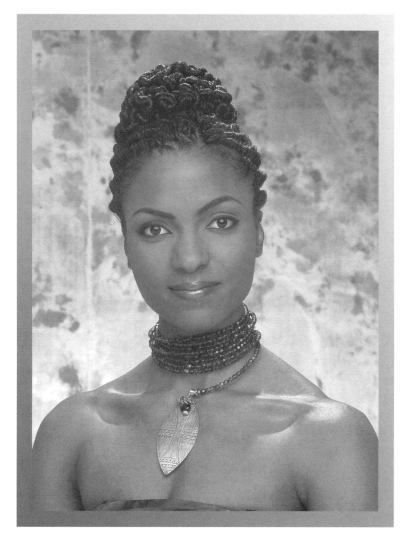

Finished style

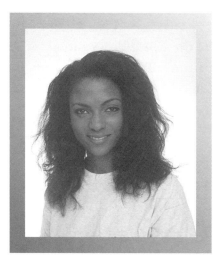

Before

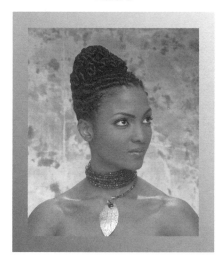

Silk twist—finished, side

This flat twist is stately and majestic and is featured by master braider N'gone Sow of Soween Braids in New York. The silky twist is intricate yet quick and easy. This style was created by laying the synthetic hair or lin flat onto equal portions of natural hair. The hair was parted into sections about the size of a large cornrow base.

A roll-twist motion secures the fiber. This pre-planned design is parted into a sculpted updo and rolled in the back. The extension chignon on top is gelled, pinned, and then sewn to secure the rolled and looped strands.

This rolled twist requires little maintenance. The client must oil the scalp once or twice per week and cover the braided style nightly.

Silky Wrap

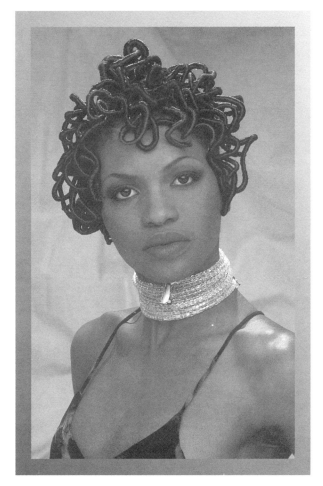

Silky wrap

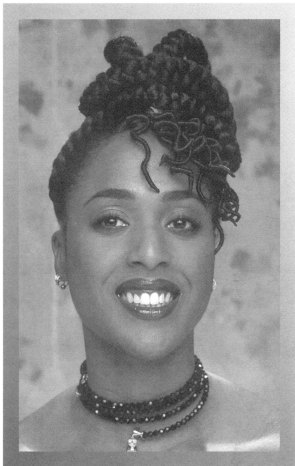

Goddess braid/silky wrap

The silky wrap is an exotic and intricate braid style. This style, mastered by freelance hair designer Susan Hale of New York, is created with synthetic hair. First, the hair is braided into a desired length and is then wrapped with an extended strip of hair. This wrapping of synthetic hair gives the braid its glossy look. Excessive winding can be uncomfortable; be aware of the stress around the hairline. After the wrapping process, the braid can be molded and shaped. Ends are singed closed. This style may last up to two months.

Silky Wrap & Goddess Braids

This combination of braid techniques is alluring and provocative. The large inverted Goddess braid lays flat on the scalp in a pre-designed sculpted pattern. Cecelia Hinds of Uzuri Braids creates this style. The extended braid is swept to the crown giving it height and dimension. The silk wrap frames the face and tendril over one eye.

NATURAL TEXTURE STYLE OPTIONS

Afros, Coil-twists, Locks

The current popularity of chemical-free, natural, or virgin hair is no fad, but is a movement toward redefining what is beautiful, acceptable, and emotionally rewarding for people with textured hair. The vicious cycle of relaxing-braiding-relaxing has stopped for many women. Today there is an opportunity for the frustrated client to be educated and offered alternative styles. As a professional braider, natural stylist, barber, or locktician, it is your responsibility to create the various options that are now mainstream fashion statements.

Remember: Everything we do is a statement about self. From what we eat to how we wear our hair, how we see and feel about ourselves is reflected. The world will have its own definition about that reflection but you must be clear and have convictions that make up your inner being—your soul.

The natural care hair specialist can be a liberator of souls. By helping clients to redefine how they see themselves, giving them more options to beauty enhancement products, and reinforcing the styling options with nurturing regular support, your clients' emotional and spiritual energy will become healthier and more vital. A new life force emerges. The client is free from stereotypical hairstyles and can just be. This empowers and builds self-esteem.

Katherine Jones, president of IBN (International Braiders Network), during a phone interview with the author, agrees: "The one word that natural hair care clients use unanimously to describe the many advantages to natural hair styles is ... freedom! Freedom to think about and participate in a variety of rewarding activities because they are no longer chained to their hair. When a woman is at peace with her hair, she is at peace with herself and the world."

Braids and extensions are a large part of African history. Today, these traditional African hair care methods have re-emerged as an essential component to bringing one closer to one's natural hair. Extensions are transitional in that they are a means to maintain one's natural hair.

After the client has worn braids for several years, the most basic step would be to remove the extensions and "go natural." This means that the client is ready to welcome and surrender to their texture, kink, nap, or coil. The natural hair care specialist can help the client to change perspective and accept genetic inheritance.

There are Afros, coil-twists, and the ultimate of natural hair—the lock. Variations of these styles are endless and, for the future, we will see men and women opting to wear these textured styles. It does not matter whether the client's hair is textured or not; the redefining of our cultural aesthetics frees everyone, even those stylists that define beauty with more European standards.

The following natural styles offer the client an opportunity to finally accept their hair.

Blow Out

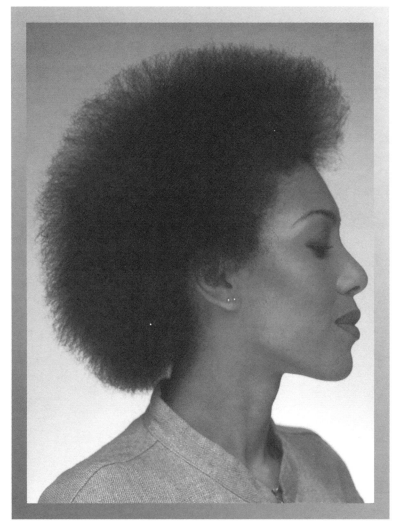

Finished style

The "blow out" is a blown dried Afro. The heat from the blow dryer elongates the hair giving it a longer, fuller look. Avoid excessive heat and pulling when blow drying.

STEP 1

After hair is blown dry, divide the hair into four to six sections from the nape of the neck to the occipital bone. Hair clip or twist away to separate sections.

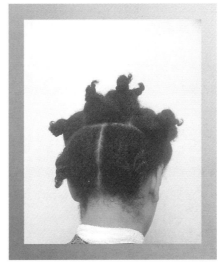

Divide hair into 4 to 6 sections.

STEP 2

To trim ends 1/4 ", use the first section as a guide. Hold a 1" subsection down with hand in line with horizontal parting. Cut to the desired length. This establishes your design guide line.

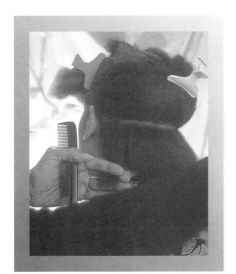

Establish guide line.

STEP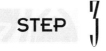

Move up the head and part off a 1/2" vertical section. Bring first guide line into this vertical section, connect lengths and cut. This creates the design for the length side. Continue upward after every new section for the desired look.

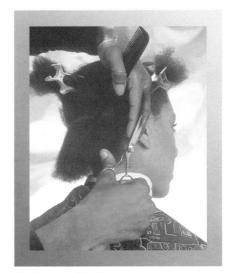

Vertical guide line

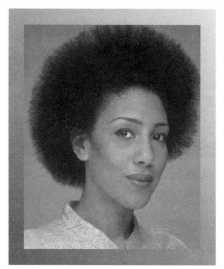

Classic blow out—finished style

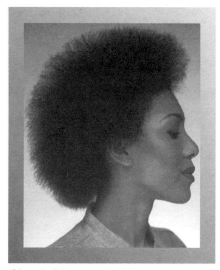

Classic blow out (side)

STEP 4

To create uniform layers with textured hair, use guide lines to maintain shape and length. For the top, hold the 1" section at a 90 degree angle (straight up) and cut straight across. Comb into the sides and the back guide line and connect lengths.

STEP 5

Use a pick or large-tooth comb to comb out hair. Comb or pick to make sure hair is distributed evenly. Stand back and observe your work from a distance; make certain the weight of the hair is properly distributed for the desired style.

STEP 6

Repeat the procedure until the cut is entirely even. Spray with oil sheen to finish the style.

The African Kurl (Twist Out)

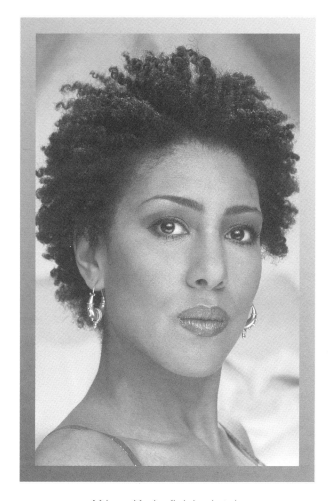

African Kurl—finished style

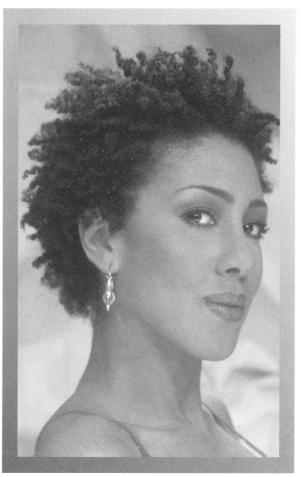

African Kurl (side)

The basic "blow out" previously shown was transformed into textured tresses that can be worn at the office, or for an evening out. It softly flows and bounces to all the urban beats.

The African Kurl is wonderful because it can be offered as a service for more than one style.

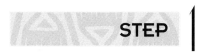

STEP 1

The hair is double twisted on the individual braid pattern. This is a double twist set—the hair is wet and sprayed with a setting lotion.

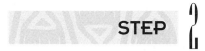

STEP 2

After the hair is totally dry, the client can wear this twist style for two or three weeks. Oil the scalp sparingly once or twice a week.

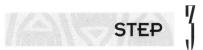

STEP 3

After a week or two, if the client wants to change the style, offer to un-twist the twists. We call it "twist out." The "twist out" can be done on the same day of the set for a beautiful, fresh look. Some clients opt to wait one to two weeks before opening the twist in order to add versatility and long life to the crimped tresses.

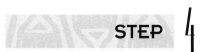

STEP 4

Separate each twist for a full, bountiful look. Avoid disturbing the wave pattern. Use fingers to fan out the twist. A small pick can be used to remove parts and to lift. Only use a pick at the base of the scalp. This will last two to three weeks. Use moisturizing sheen when necessary.

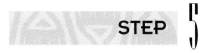

STEP 5

This set can also be applied to relaxed, straight hair. Drying time is one hour and perm rods can be used for a spiral, fuller effect.

The Short Afro

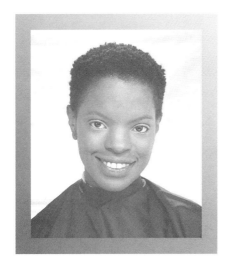

Before

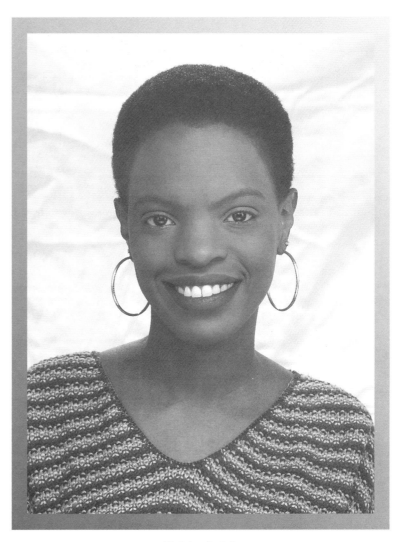

Finished style

The short Afro for women is created by a free form of cutting curly hair using a clipper and a large comb. The hair is graduated from the perimeter up and is cut to work with the head shape. Naeemah Jeff of 'Locks' N Chops' Natural Hair Salon in New York uses the following technique, in which the hair is cut when it is dry.

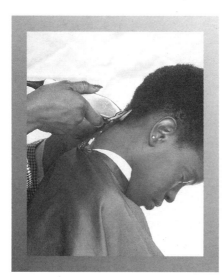

Cut the first quarter inch.

STEP 1

First pick the hair out, using a jumbo comb with wide-set teeth. Observe its density closely—particularly if your client does not want much of the scalp to show through. Extremely curly hair gives the illusion that it is cut close, you will not see the scalp, but density counts most when deciding how close to cut the hair. In this instance, based on the client's desires, only the first 1/2" at the nape and sides is cut so close that some of the scalp shows through.

STEP 2

Begin at the nape and have the client lean forward with her chin resting on her chest. Cut the first 1/4", using a clipper-over-comb technique. Place the comb flat against the head.

STEP 3

Move to the next section, smoothly bringing the comb upward and cutting again. Observe the first 1/2" to make certain that the hair is as close or as far away from the scalp as you want it.

STEP 4

Continue cutting in this manner, working with the head shape. About 1" up the head, begin graduating the cut. Use the angle of the comb to do this. Angle the comb slightly away from the head as you cut, and continue working up the back of the head. Rotate the tips of the comb toward the head as you lift the hair to create graduation. Work with a smooth, flowing motion, inserting the comb and working across sections, then moving up. (Avoid jerky movements.)

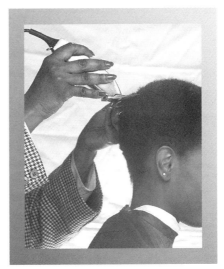

Angle the comb and cut.

STEP 5

When you reach the occipital, stand back and observe your work at a distance to make certain the weight is properly distributed. (If you observe your work from too close a vantage point, you could be fooled into thinking the shape is cleaner than it actually is.)

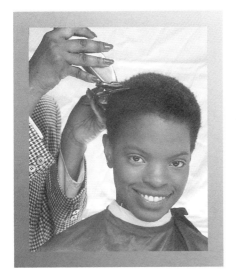

Graduate the hair.

STEP 6

Next move to the sides and repeat this procedure to cut the first 1/2" or so very close to the head. Then angle the comb to graduate the hair and work to the top of the head. Repeat this procedure on the opposite side.

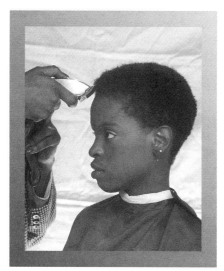

Cut the front hairline.

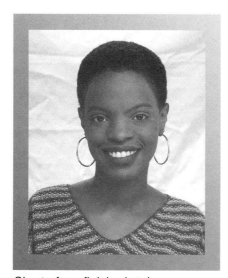

Short afro—finished style

STEP 7

To complete the cut, lift the front hairline and cut it freehand with the clippers. Then dampen the dry hair and add a liquid polish styling product.

African Kurl and Flat Twist "Sunburst"

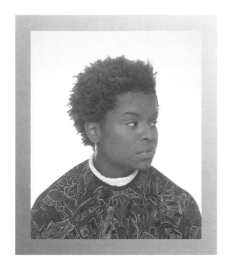

Before

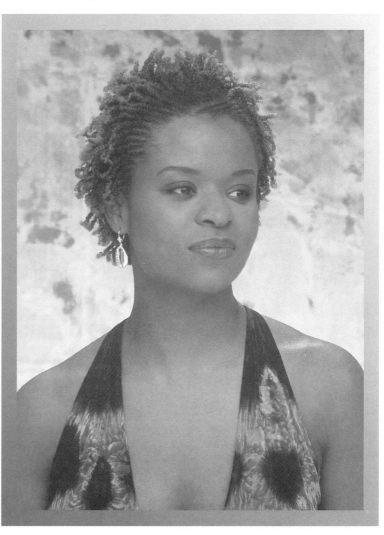

Finished style

This combination of natural twist is fresh and youthful. The styles mix a curly look with the sculpted flat twist that spreads sunshine to every face. The tighter the coil pattern, the more texture the curls will have. These curls are versatile and can last for up to six weeks.

For more fullness and volume, a twist out service can be offered. The stylist can un-twist both the kurls and the flat twist for styling options.

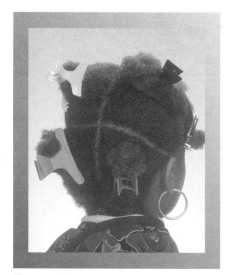

Four sections

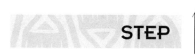
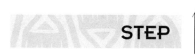

STEP 1

Shampoo and deep condition the hair. Towel dry, squeezing out excess moisture. Hair should be damp but not dripping wet.

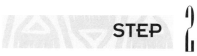

STEP 2

With tail comb, divide the hair in half from ear to ear. Then divide the back portion of the hair into four sections.

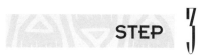

STEP 3

Begining at the nape, lightly apply a pinch of water-soluble gel to each subsection. With a horizontal parting, sub-divide vertically 1/4" partings. Overlap equal portions counter-clockwise and two-strand twist to the ends of the strand. The twist must be tight, so revolutions should be close together to form the curl pattern.

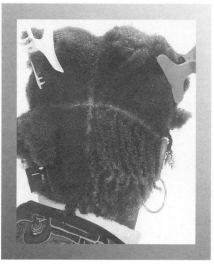

Close together to form curl.

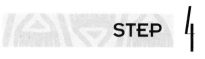

STEP 4

When the back is completed, move to the side and repeat the twist movement.

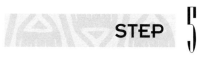

STEP 5

Dampen hair in front with a spray bottle of water and oil to keep moist. Flat twist damp hair into a small, sculpted pattern. Place under dryer until completely dry.

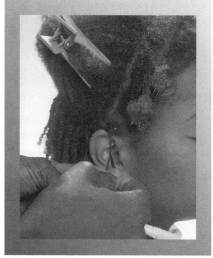

Lower side two strands.

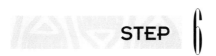

STEP 6

Lightly oil scalp and finish with moisturizing spray sheen.

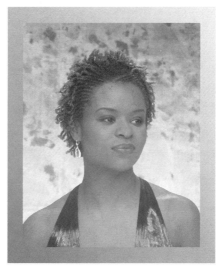

Sunburst twist—finished style

NUBIAN COILS

Styling the hair in Nubian coils is the first step toward locking hair. Nubian coils are small spiral formed curls usually short to medium in length. The texture of the hair determines the formation or coil pattern. Some coil patterns are tighter or closer together than others. If the coil pattern is smaller, then the coil will be tight. The reverse also holds true: the larger the wave or curl formation, the larger in size the actual coil will be. By examining the coil pattern of several strands of hair over the entire head, the stylist will be able to determine the size and characteristics of the coil formation.

Conduct a brief consultation to examine the client's hair for coil pattern. Check three different areas of the head:

1. *The nape (the "kitchen") is usually tight, very coily or curly, and dense.*

2. *The side hairline usually slightly less coily or curly and may be thinner or finer in density. Look for damage or alopecia.*

3. *The crown may have the least curl or wave pattern. For some menopausal women, this area may thin and bald. However, this area is usually rich with a dense capacity of hair.*

The average client has several textures of hair from grey wiry to fine coily. What this means is that the stylist must be aware of the differences and apply the necessary techniques based on the hair texture to get the best results before locking.

Nubian coils are the "pre-lock phase" before African locks or dread locks, as they are often called. This pre-locked phase is a beautiful style in itself and can be worn to work or for play. It is neat yet at the same time loose in structure. When done initially, Nubian coils are flat and contoured to the head. By using different styling gels, a shiny/glossy glow gives the coils their finished look. However, after about forty-eight hours, the coil "puffs" open slightly—just enough to expand the spiral and soften the curl. The coil formation is still in place and can last for up to six weeks. The life of this coiled style depends on the size of the coil. Smaller coils last longer and the tighter the coil or curl pattern the longer the style will last since this style is the preparatory style for African locks.

During the consultation, it is necessary that the stylist know whether the client intends to lock or just wants to wear his or her hair in a natural coiled style. The person that is interested in locking is at a higher commitment level, physically, emotionally and spiritually willing to invest the time—which is usually six months to a year—for the locks to solidify and mature.

Hair locking is a natural coiling process of textured curly hair without the use of combs or chemicals. The hair meshes and spirals within itself, interlocking and adhering until the joined strands become a tight, dense unit or lock. The hair locks in slow developmental stages, which can take anywhere from six months to a year depending on the length, density, and coil pattern. Cultivating locks is a process, a journey into self discovery and acceptance of our genetic and cultural inheritance.

There are several ways to cultivate locks such as double twisting, wrapping with cord or wire braiding with or without extension, or simply not disturbing the hair by not combing or brushing the lock (like the Rastafarians of Jamaica do)—by just leaving the hair to its own natural course, the hair will lock. However, it will not have a groomed, manicured look. I refer to these type of locks as "organic" locks. Cultivated African locks have symmetry and balance. The goal to grooming locks is to create uniformed tresses that will turn heads when the client is well groomed. Symmetry is not easy to accomplish with textured hair. Although the hair is programmed genetically to coil, no two coils are exactly alike. It is the locktician's or natural hair care stylist's responsibility to develop a system that promotes symmetry into the textured hair. Three basic methods of locking are: (1) comb technique; (2) palm roll and (3) braid or extension.

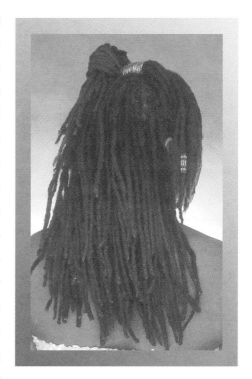

Mature locks

The most effective techniques that use the natural coil pattern are the comb technique and the palm roll method. The comb technique can be most effective during the early stages of locking while the coil is still open. This method of coiling entails placing the comb at the base and, in a rotating motion, spiraling the hair into a curl. With each revolution the comb moves down until it reaches the end of the hair shaft. It offers a great tight coil and is excellent on short (1 to 3") hair.

The second method of grooming and starting locks is the palm roll method. This method is the gentlest on the hair and guides it through all the natural stages of locking. Palm rolling takes advantage of the hair's natural ability to coil. The following description shows how to use the palm roll method to create a coiled style.

Nubian coils— Pre-Locking Phase

STEP 1

To begin, shampoo and condition the hair. Then towel blot the hair, squeezing out excess moisture so that the hair is damp but not wet.

STEP 2

Next part the hair in horizontal rows from the nape all the way to the front hairline. Then divide the first horizontal row at the nape into equal-sized subsections. The subsections can be square, circular, triangular, or rectangular; the size of the individual sections and their shape depends on the client's desired finished look. Before palm rolling, use the hair clips to hold the hair around the subsection out of the way.

STEP 3

Beginning at the nape on the far side, take the hair within the first subsection and lightly apply a pinch of gel, using your right forefinger and thumb. Then pinch the hair near the scalp and twist it one full counter-clockwise revolution. (If you are left-handed, use your left hand to pinch the hair, but always turn it counter-clockwise.)

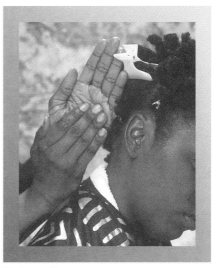

Palm rolling

STEP 4

With one smooth motion, pass the hair from your right hand to your left hand, tuck the hair into the recession near the thumb and fold your thumb down to hold the hair in place. Position your left hand behind your right hand so that the left fingertips are at the right wrist. Slide your right hand back while simultaneously sliding the hand forward.

STEP 5

When the hair is between your palms, pull out your thumb so that the hair is rolled between your palms. When the fingertips of your right hand are near the left-hand wrist, fold your thumb back down to recapture the hair.

STEP 6

So that the hair is always rolled in a counter-clockwise direction, reposition the left hand behind the right hand and repeat the palm rolling technique. Each time you roll the hair, move progressively down the hair shaft. When you reach the ends, place the lock down neatly and begin again with the adjacent subsection.

STEP 7

When each subsection in the first horizontal row has been completed, move up to the next horizontal row and subdivide it as before. If you rolled the previous subsections from right to left, this time work from left to right. Continue this pattern all the way to the crown. As you work up the head, include the side sections. Always maintain a degree of moisture by using the spray bottle as needed. Also, apply the same amount of gel to each subsection.

STEP 8

When you reach the crown, continue palm rolling subsections, directing them to move toward the back. When you reach the top of the head, move around the client to accommodate the desired finished style. If the client wants the front individualized, for instance, if a few sections are to move onto the forehead, reposition yourself in front of of the client to palm roll these subsections.

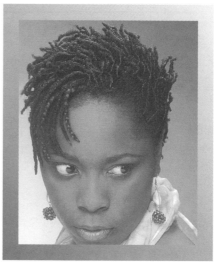

Nubian coils with yarn extension

STEP 9

When all the hair has been palm rolled, place the client under a hood dryer set on low heat. Dry the hair completely, but no more than necessary.

STEP 10

When the hair is completely dry, finish the style by applying a light oil to add sheen.

STEP 11

Single braids with yarn are a lock alternative which is added to the front to frame the face. The ends are looped and singed to the desired length.

AFRICAN LOCKS

The ultimate in natural hair care is the textured richness of hair locking. Throughout the continent of Africa various tribes have practiced this art form and cultural expression of beauty enhancement. The people of the Pokot, Massai, Mau Mau, Kau, Ashanti, and Fulani, as well as many others, practice some form of locking. Some tribes use mud or a red clay with straw or hay to perform the grooming technique.

Locks symbolize what the Afro was in the 1960s: a symbol of freedom, cultural empowerment, and identity as well as a seed to self-acceptance. Ona Osirio-Maat, a locktician for eleven years, is the creator of the **LockSmyth method**, a lock technique that incorporates a special, rhythmical palm rolling technique. Osirio-Maat states during a phone interview with the author, "Locked hair is the ultimate natural hair statement. It says you have come home... finally. The self-love and appreciation that has been gained from 'growing' through the process can have tremendous transformative power surrounding the 'locker' life. People usually undergo some deeper level of self-evaluation as they return for professional cultivation of their locks, and the stories center around their hair getting longer and stronger. Also, there are stories about the strength their locks silently display. As a locktician, I witness the internal growth of my clients as well as the inches of hair flowing down their backs. Their pride is tempered by the humility of the process. Instead of running fast, hard and long distances from the kink, they changed their perspective and began to embrace the coil."

THE DEVELOPMENTAL STAGES OF HAIR LOCKING

Depending on the coil pattern, density, and length of hair, the locking process may vary from six to twelve months to lock the entire head.

Phase I. Pre-Lock Stage—Hair is soft and is coiled into spiral configurations. The coil is smooth and the end is open. The coil has a shiny or a glossy texture.

Phase II. Sprouting Stage—Hair begins to interlace and mesh. The separate units begin to "puff up" and expand in size. The units are no longer glossy, thin, and smooth. Little bulbs or knots form at the middle or ends of the coiled unit indicating that the coil is starting to close. This "plumping" of the lock may give the head an unkempt look. Avoid over-grooming or excessive twisting at this phase. The length starts to shrink because the coil is solidifying. This "frizzy" look is part of the process. Here is where patience and desire are a virtue—and the client's level of commitment is tested. This is also the stage in which some sections of the head will be totally locked while other portions of the head will still have soft and open coils. Be aware of the different coil patterns and density of the hair in these specific areas.

      Phase III. Growing Stage—The hair strands adhere to one another, creating a network of tresses within each coiled unit. Interlacing and meshing can be felt by squeezing the lock. The stylist can feel a bulb at the end of each lock. The locking process starts at the middle or ends of the unit, not at the scalp. Hair begins to regain length. The lock still may be frizzy yet solid in some areas. Locks are closed at the ends, dense, and dull, not reflecting light to get any sheen.

Textured curly, coily hair does not reflect light the way straight hair does. The client may complain about the dullness or the lack of luster. Again, this is part of the process. Reassure the client that this perceived dullness is what creates the lock. One can add oils which allow the light to reflect off the oils and give the hair a gloss.

      Phase IV. Maturation Stage—The lock is now totally closed at the end. The unit is interlaced and meshed and in contrast to the size, giving the hair a tighter, rope-like look except where there is new growth at the base. The network of intertwined strands is tight and hard to the touch. The hair grows at a rapid rate. Whether the strands are in the **anagen cycle** or **telogen** cycle of growth, all the hair is fused together; because the hair is not combed or brushed, there is little shedding. The hair stays within the locked unit. New sprouts spring up between mature locks. In some cases, the hair forms whole new locks.

N
O
T
E
S

Some textures will not close at the end. A single curl or wave may exist at the end of the lock, giving the lock the appearance of being open. The maturation stage will still continue.

Phase V. Atrophy Stage—After several years of maturation (the usual time varies between seven and ten years) the lock may start to weaken or atrophy at the ends. The smaller the lock, the more fragile and more likely the atrophy will occur. The larger the lock, the more durable it is and the degeneration may never occur. This atrophy stage usually occurs at the nape of the neck and around the frontal and peripheral hairlines. When the client's hair starts to weaken, consult and make sure it is part of a natural locking process and not due to physical or emotional stress. How to tell the difference:

1. *Thinning and breakage at the ends is a degenerative process and part of the locks' life cycle; excessive dryness and texture can accelerate this process.*

2. *Thinning and breakage at the base or scalp is the body's warning signal that something is internally or externally imbalanced.*

HOW TO CULTIVATE AND GROOM LOCKS

There is an effective seven-step procedure for grooming and cultivating locks:

1. *To start locks, use the palm roll technique described earlier in the chapter.*

2. *Avoid over-twisting. With each revolution move down the shaft to avoid over-spiraling the hair.*

3. *During the first three months, the client should return to the stylist every three or four weeks to have the locks groomed.*

4. *Grooming may entail:*

   - *herbal shampoo*
   - *hot oil treatment*
   - *herbal rinse or acid rinse*
   - *re-rolling, cultivating, or manicuring*
   - *trim (optional)*
   - *styling (texturizing to include crimping, curling, braiding, and so on)*
   - *watering: spritzing locks with water helps keep locks or natural curls clean. The weight of water helps the lock drop down in length and brings lint to the surface. Keeping it wet is one of the keys to lock growth and promotes the natural curling of hair.*

5. *Always remove lock debris, lint, and excess oils embedded in locks.*

6. *Avoid using heavy petroleum or waxy oils. Use diluted moisturizing and water-soluble gels when rolling the hair.*

7. *Once the locks are fully matured, the client's hair can be shampooed more often.*

Be careful not to dry out the hair. Use lemon rinses and acid rinses to loosen the lock debris after each shampoo for deep cleansing. Follow with light, hot oil treatments to the scalp.

Locked hair may appear dull, lackluster, or drab when not properly cared for. Locks do, however, have a beautiful sheen and luster when healthy and clean. The sheen is subtly understated and soft because, like most natural fibers, locks have a matte finish; this finish is a part of their natural beauty and uniqueness. Avoid applying large amounts of braid oil or moisturizing sheen to create more shine; this contributes to lock sediment build-up. Once or twice a week small amounts of natural oil (dime-size) can be applied to the scalp and massaged through the hair to create luster. With locks, "less is more."

STYLING AND TEXTURIZING LOCKS

At the salon Tendrils in Brooklyn, NY, texture is used to enhance the natural tress. The finer the lock, the more versatility the stylist will have to create new looks. Avoid putting too much stress on the hair to eliminate breakage. Remember: Thin locks are fragile.

> *Texturizing—On damp locks, lightly spray a setting lotion. Braid or twist the entire length. Add a perm rod or clip to hold the end. The hair must be completely dry before unbraiding or twisting out in order to get style.*

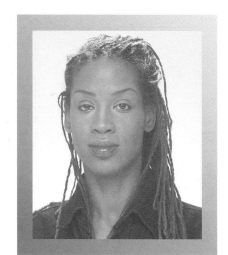

Before

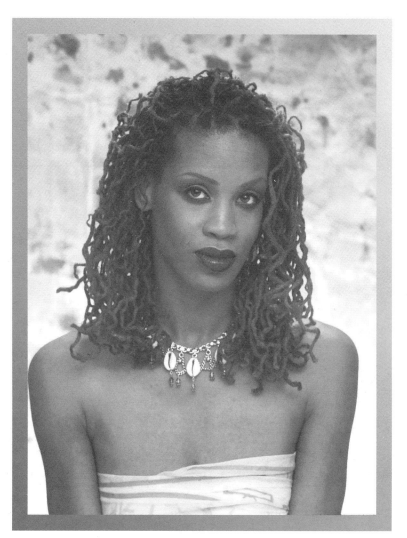

Finished style

🗲 *Tendrils/Spirals—On damp locks, lightly spray a setting lotion to the entire lock surface. With a perm rod (pink, purple, or white), vertically wind the lock around the rod, starting at the end of the hair and moving up toward the scalp.*

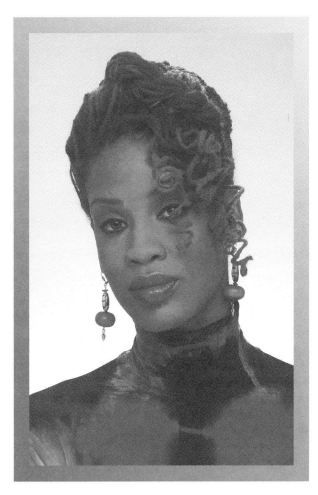

Upswept locks—spiral curl

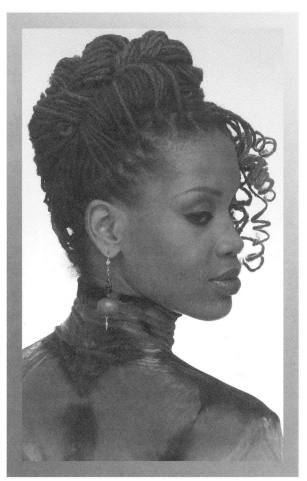

Upswept locks—side

Updo Sweeps—Roll, twist, braid, pin, and tuck. Create chignons, buns, french rolls, and inverted braids—be as creative as your hair will let you. There are no limits!

MATERIALS FOR EXTENSIONS

There are a variety of materials that are available for the purpose of extending textured hair. The life of the style, however, will always be determined by the materials used. As braid extensions become more popular, more varieties of quality and price will be available. Though it may save money to buy the least expensive product, especially if you buy in large quantities, beware that you may not get the desired results. In other words, the extension material is critical to the final outcome of your hair design.

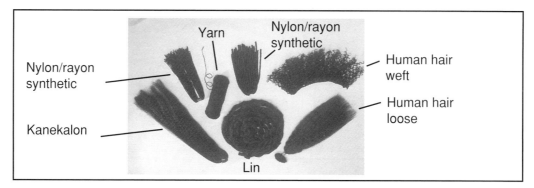

Figure 10.1   Extension materials

When buying a new product, buy in small quantities and test the fiber on a mannequin before using it on a client.

The following list may help you to decide what extension material to use:

1. *Kanekalon—It is a manufactured synthetic fiber of excellent quality. It is designed to have a texture similar to African hair types. It does not reflect light, which means it has less shine. It is durable and holds up to shampooing and styling. When braiding the hair, it is smooth to the scalp and fingers which is very important because it does not cut or damage natural hair as other less expensive products do. It generally has a softer feel and tangles less than other synthetics. It comes in a variety of colors. It is versatile and easy to match with natural hair colors. Kanekalon costs more than most synthetics but is a better quality—not only according to manufacturers but also according to many braid stylists. This extension material finishes well when using the singeing method; it burns safely and seals quickly.*

2. *Nylon/Rayon Synthetic—This product is less expensive and readily available. The quality can vary depending on the brand name. You must be familiar with the brands in order to get a decent quality. In general, the less expensive synthetic hair tangles more and can damage natural hair. Nylon and rayon have been known to cut or break the hair. They are often less durable after repeated shampooing. They also reflect light and leave hair very shiny.*

It has been my experience that when the hair is shampooed regularly, the natural hair begins to expand—but the kanekalon or synthetic hair does not. As the natural hair expands, the tension at the base of the braid with the extension increases.

Warning: This extension material finishes poorly when using the singeing method; melted fibers can stick to the skin and burn. Avoid this material when singeing.

Stylists must be cautious when choosing the quality of the extension material. Nylon and rayon synthetics, however, come in more varieties of color than Kanekalon. However, these materials do not burn well when using the singe method to close synthetic extensions. The warm plastic melts too quickly, holds heat, and can burn and blister the client's skin.

3. *Human Hair—This material is the most confusing of fibers and is somewhat mysterious. Most of the product is imported from Asia. It is a closed market, and very little is known abut how the human hair is produced or processed. Some of it is imported from Europe and small amounts are from Africa. Although the label may say human hair, buyer beware—all that glitters is not gold. The buyer must select hair from a reputable dealer or a wholesaler of this product to be assured of*

its quality. Pre-packaged human hair is generally less expensive than that which is customized by a wholesaler. If a wholesaler is not available in your area, consider mail order.

This material (supposedly) is derived from human hair and is processed into hundreds of colors and textures. It is versatile, soft, and tangle free. Although the material is extremely expensive, sometimes overpriced, it moves and feels like natural hair. It expands along with human hair when it is washed, which may also change the desired results and the life of a particular hairstyle. It can easily slip from the base of the braid. But unlike Kanekalon, it can be reused, if properly cleaned and combed. This product is ideal for those who are allergic to the synthetic products. To finish braid styles with human hair you can use thermal curling tools and set the hair for crimps.

4. *Human Hair Weft—Wefted human hair has all the advantages of loose human hair, except that when it is shampooed it does not expand to the point that it can slip from the base. The material is sewn together on a woven strip that interlaces the individual human hair strands. Wefted human hair is a great alternative to add dimension, length, and color to a client's natural hair. Wefted hair is sewn in with a needle and thread to a braided cornrow track and netting.*

5. *Yarn—Traditional yarn material is used to make fabric for sweaters, hats, and so on. But now it is being used to adorn textured African hair. When braided or wrapped, it is light, soft, and detangles easily. Yarn comes in many colors. The most commonly used is black or brown for a more natural look. It is different than synthetic fibers because it does not reflect any light. It is not glossy. It gives the braid style a matte finish and can give braids a "locked" look. But be careful when choosing yarns. Some black yarns have a blue or green tint. A yarn may appear jet black in the store but in the light it reflects green. Always hold yarn to the light before purchasing. It is very inexpensive and easy to find. Also, the yarn can be cotton or a nylon blend and though it may expand when shampooing, it does not slip from the base. So, braid styles are durable with yarns. Do not burn yarns if they are 100% cotton. Finish braids with a neat knot.*

6. *Lin—This is a beautiful wool fiber made in France and imported from Africa. Like yarn, it has a matte finish and gives off little shine. It only comes in black and brown. Lin can be pur-*

chased in packages of 25 meters or 24 yards. It comes on a roll and is used in any length and size. Often used for Senegalese twists and "Corkscrew" styles, this fiber cannot be singed. It is cottony and very flammable. Braid styles using lin are generally not shampooed often.

7. *Yak— This strong textured fiber comes from the domestic ox, usually found in the mountains of Tibet and Central Asia. The hairs on the ox are long on the sides and the back. These hairs are shaven and processed to use alone or blended with human hair. The variety of blends usually creates a more African texture when yak is used in wigs. Small mixtures of yak with human hair helps to remove the manufactured shine. (See Fig 10.1 for pictures of these materials.)*

BIBLIOGRAPHY

Afrika, Dr. Llaila C. *African Holistic Health*. Brooklyn, New York: A & B Books Publishers, 1993.

Airola, Dr. Paavo. *Stop Hair Loss*. Phoenix, Arizona: Health Publishing, 1984.

Balch, C.N.C. Phyllis & Balch, Dr. James. *Prescription for Cooking and Dietary Wellness*. Greenfield, Indiana: P.A.B. Publishing, 1993.

Begoun, Paula. *Don't Go Shopping For Hair Care Products Without Me*. Seattle, Washington: Beginning Press, 1995.

Chesky, Sheldon R., Cristina, Isabel and Rosenberg, Richard B. *Playing It Safe: Milady's Guide to Decontamination, Sterilization, and Personal Protection*. Albany, New York: Milady Publishing, 1994.

Evans, Nekhena. *Everything You Need to Know About Hairlocking*. Brooklyn, New York: New Bein' Press, 1993.

Ferrell, Pam. *Where Beauty Touches Me*. Washington, DC: Cornrows & Co. Publication, 1993.

Haigh, Rachel. *The Neal's Yard Bakery Wholefood Cook Book*. Topsfield, Massachusetts: Salem House Publishers, 1986.

Hampton, Aubrey. *Natural Organic Hair and Skin Care*. Tampa, Florida: Organica Press, 1984.

Hoffman, David. *The New Holistic Herbal*. New York: Barnes & Noble Books, 1990.

Keller, Erick. *Aromatherapy Handbook for Beauty, Hair and Skin Care*. Rochester, Vermont: Healing Arts Press, 1991.

Kowalchik & Hylton, Ed. Rodale's *Illustrated Encyclopedia of Herbs*. Emmaus, Pennsylvania: Rodale Press Inc., 1987.

Lawless, Julia. *The Illustrated Encyclopedia of Essential Oils*. New York: Element Books/Barnes & Noble Books, 1995.

Milady's Standard Textbook of Cosmetology, Revised Edition. Albany, New York: Milady Publishing, 1995.

Morrow, Willie. *400 Years Without a Comb*. San Diego, California: Morrow's Publishing Research Development, 1990.

Olsen, Elsie. *Disorders of Hair Growth, Diagnosis and Treatment* O'Donoghue, Marianne Nelson "Hair Care Products" 1994.

Olsen, Elsie. *Disorders of Hair Growth, Diagnosis and Treatment* Wilbron, Dr. Wesley "Disorders of Hair Growth in African-Americans" 1994.

Robertson, Flinders & Ruppenthal. *Laurel's Kitchen Recipes*. Berkeley, California: Ten Speed Press, 1976.

Rose, Jeanne. *Jeanne Rose's Herbal Body Book*. New York: Grosset & Dunlap, 1976.

SalonOvations' The Multicultural Client: Cuts, Styles and Chemical Services. Albany, New York: Milady Publishing, 1995.

Schoon, Douglas. *HIV/AIDS & Hepatitis: Everything You Need to Know to Protect Yourself and Others*. Albany, New York: Milady Publishing Company, 1994.

Scoleri, Donald W. and Lascony, Dr. Lewis E. *The New Psy-Cosmetologist* Reading, PA: Salon Today Publications, 1988.

Tourles, Stephanie. *The Herbal Body Book*. Pownal, Vermont: Storey Publishing, 1994.

Waajid, Taliah *Keep Up the Roots: Hairitage, Braids & Weave Masterpieces*. College Park, Georgia: Hairitage Publications, 1995.

Whilton, Shirley. *Essential Oils & Essences*. Edison, New Jersey: Chartwell Books, 1995.

Winter, Ruth. *A Consumer's Dictionary of Cosmetic Ingredients*. New York: Crown Publishers, 1976.

Worwood, Valerie Ann. *The Complete Book of Essential Oils & Aromatherapy*. San Rafael, California: New World Library, 1991.

Zone, Guy. *The House of the Heart Is Never Full and Other Proverbs of Africa*. New York: Simon & Schuster, 1993.

INDEX

A

Acid rinses—used to neutralize or restore the pH balance (acid mantle) to the hair. 155-56 *See also* **Rinses and Tonics**

Acidic pH—the lower the number for the content on the pH scale below the optimal neutral pH level of 7 for hair. 78

Acne Keloidalis. *See* **Folliculitis Keloidalis**

Acquired canities—gray hair due to old age or the onset prematurely in early adult life. 76

Acquired Immune Deficiency Syndrome—a fatal disease caused by the human immunodeficiency virus that destroys the body's defenses against disease and infection. 30-31
protection, 31
risks, 30

Acquired immunity—a type of immunity the body develops after it has overcome a disease or through inoculation. 18

Aesthetic shampoo, 132-33

African Kurl, 182, 231-32
and Flat Twist "Sunburst", 237-39

African locks, 245

Afro, 8-9, 182, 233-36

Afro "Congo Crown", 215-17

Afro Weave, 182, 214

Aggressive communication—over-reacts to situations. 39 *See also* **Communication forms**

AIDS. *See* **Acquired Immune Deficiency Syndrome**

Alcohol, 29-30

Alkaline level—a pH higher than 7 on the pH scale for hair. 78

Almond oil, 141

Aloe vera, 26, 140-41

Alopecia—a general term describing a variety of abnormal hair loss conditions. 86-93
factors, 86
treatment, 88-89
types, 87

Alopecia areata—refers to the sudden or unrecognized falling out of hair in patches or spots; usually triggered by trauma to the nervous system and circulatory system in the lymphatic system. 87

Alopecia prematura—balding which occurs at a slow pace with a thinning process usually during middle age. 87

Alopecia senilis—loss of hair or balding that occurs with old age. 87

Ampholytes—(or amphoterics) cling to the hair making it appear more manageable; mildest of the detergents and claim not to strip the natural oils from the hair and scalp. 128-29

Anagen growth—the period of development when the bulb is moving up through the follicle. 67, 246 *See also* **Hair**, growth cycles

Animal parasitic infections, 95

Anionic—a high foaming, lots of suds, shampoo. 127

Anti-dandruff
herbs/oils, 139
products, 83

Antiseptics—sanitizers that are safe to use on the skin, scalp and hair which can reduce and kill bacteria. 26, 138

Apricot, 164

Arrector pili muscle—an involuntary muscle under the hair follicle, which allows the hair to contract, and stand up when you are afraid or shivering cold. *fig.* 5.1, 62

Aromatherapy, 88

Aromatic oils, 88

Assertive communication—reacts to situations appropriately. 39 *See also* **Communication forms**

Astringent, 140

Atrophy—hair that has stopped growing and begins to shrink and fall out excessively. 86-87, 247

Autoclave, steam—a sterilizing chamber that uses high heat and steamed pressure to kill all living organisms. 19-20

Avocado, 141, 164

B

B complex—vitamins that provide the body with energy by converting carbohydrates into glucose (sugar), which the body needs to burn in order to produce energy. 106-107

Bacilli—short rod-shaped organisms. 15 *See* **Pathogenic**

Bacteria—minute, one-celled vegetable microorganisms found nearly everywhere; also known as germs. 10
classifications, 15
entering the body, 17
infection, 16-17
life cycle, 15-16
movement, 15
shapes, 15

Bacteriology—the science that deals with the study of microorganisms called bacteria. 10

Balsam of Peru, 141-42

Balsam of Tolu, 141-42

Barbicide, 31. *See also* **Disinfectants**, types

Base relaxer. *See* **Petrolatum**

Basil, 142

Beebalm. *See* **Bergamot**

Beeswax, 142

Benzoin tincture, 26

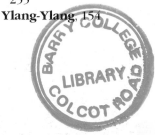

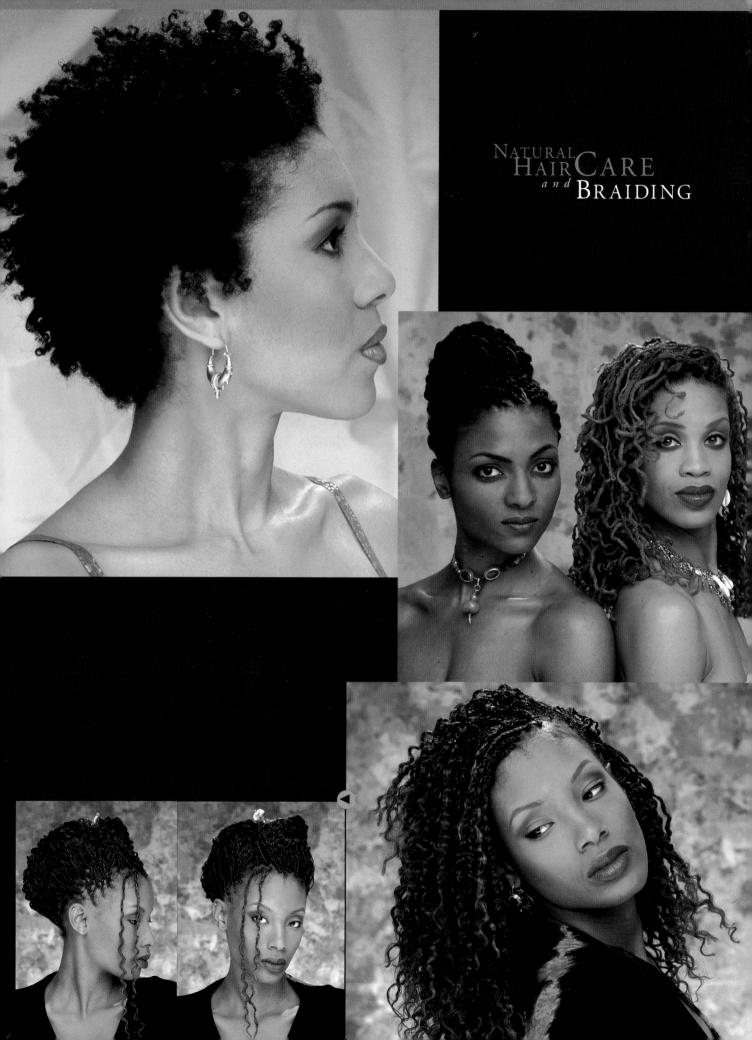

NATURAL
HAIR CARE
and
BRAIDING

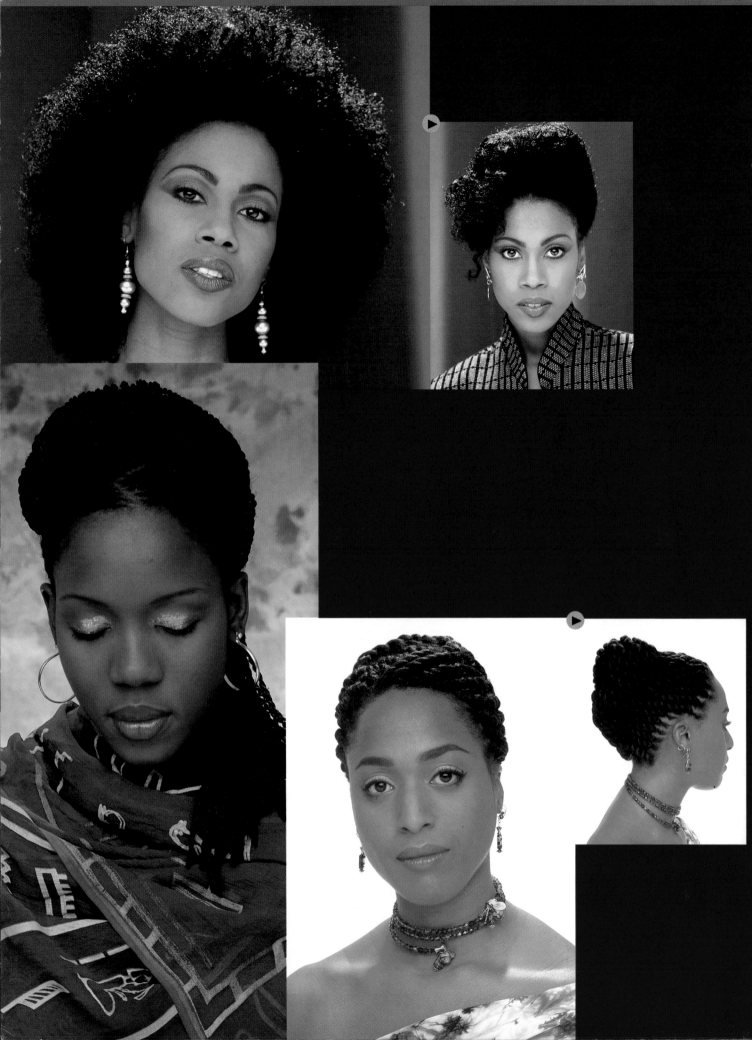

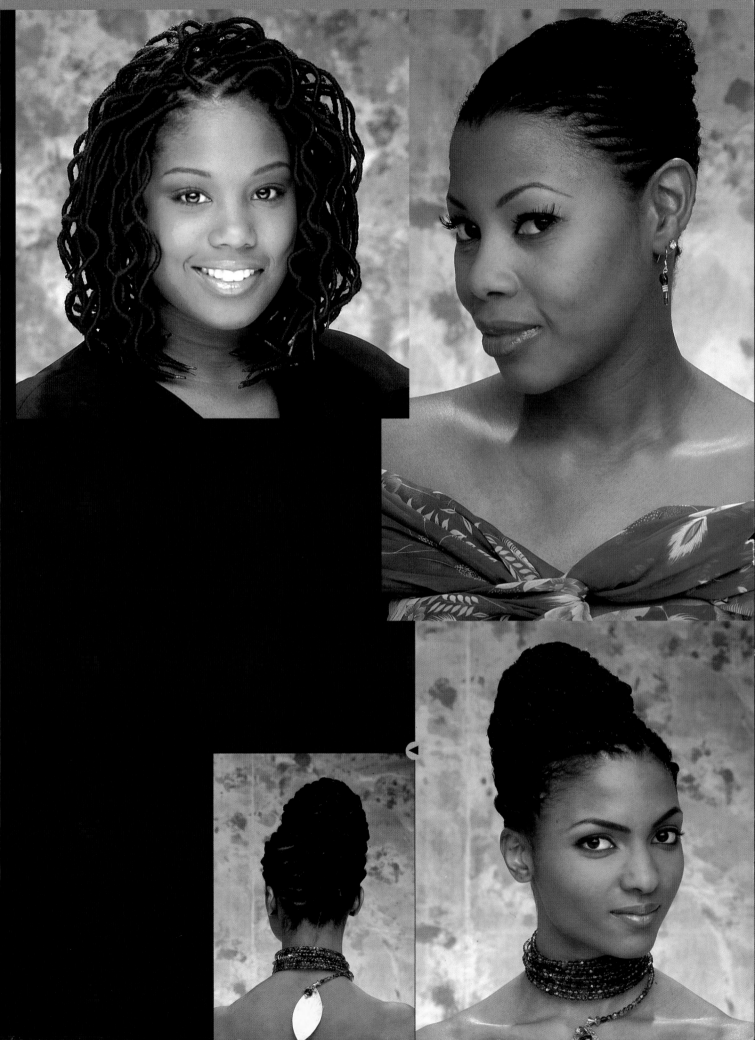

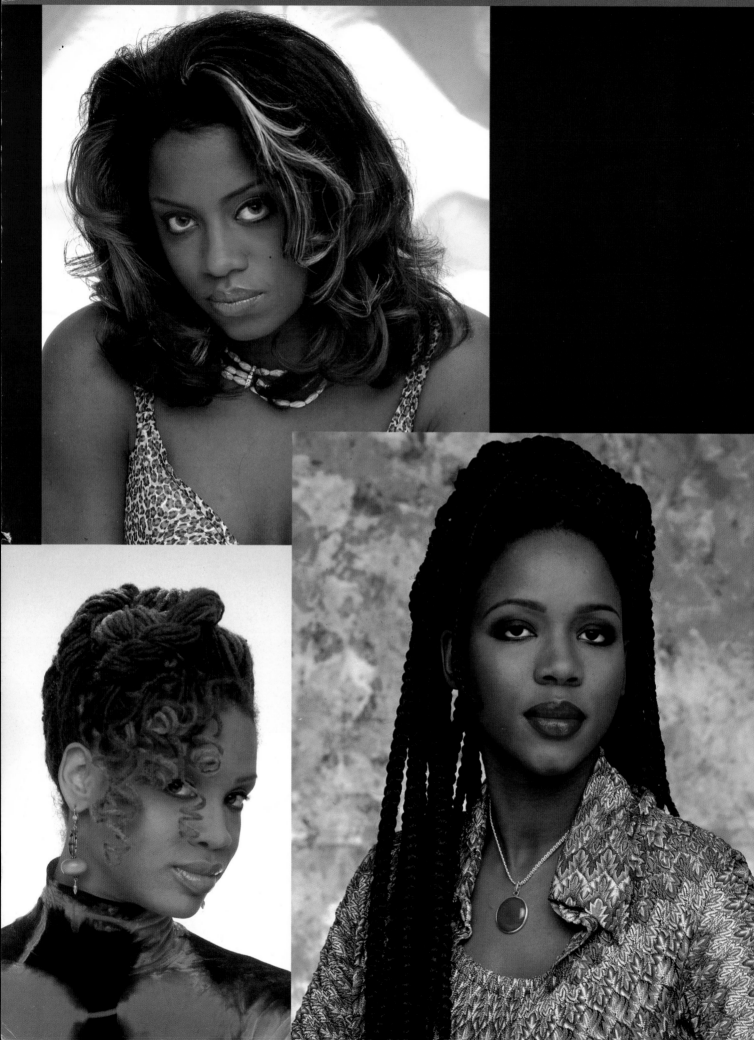

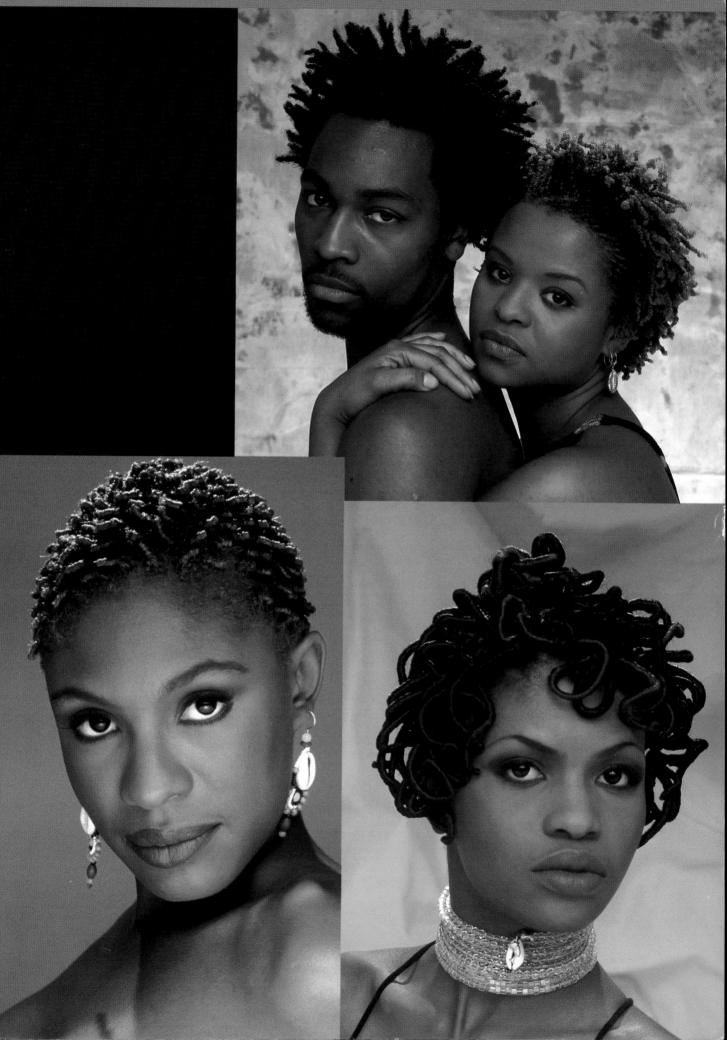

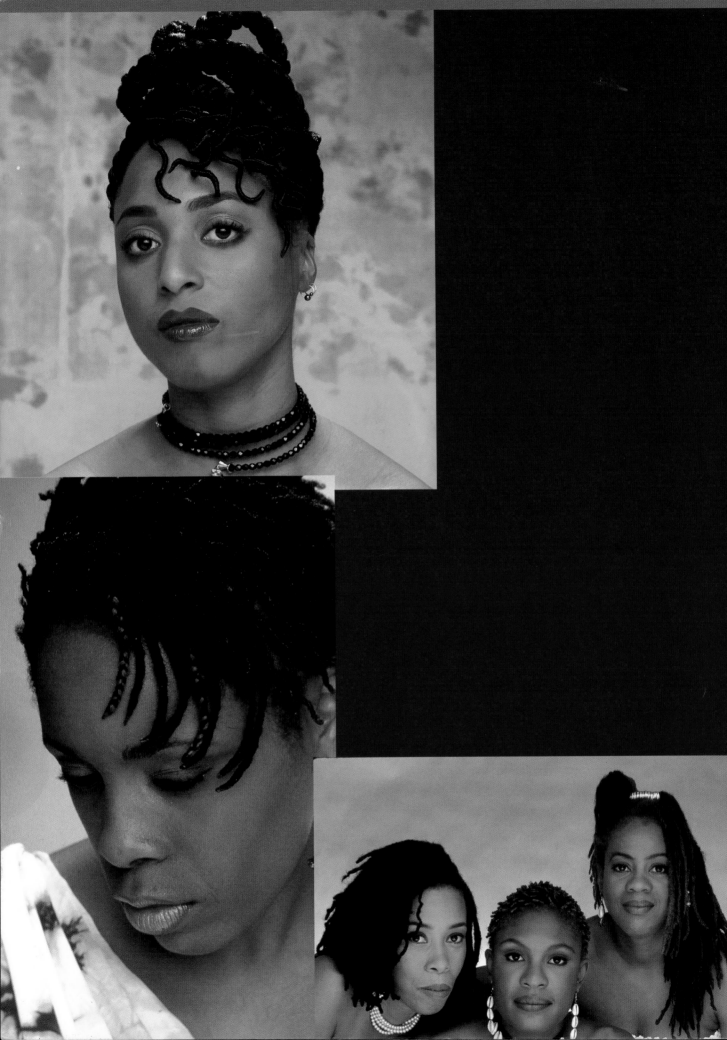

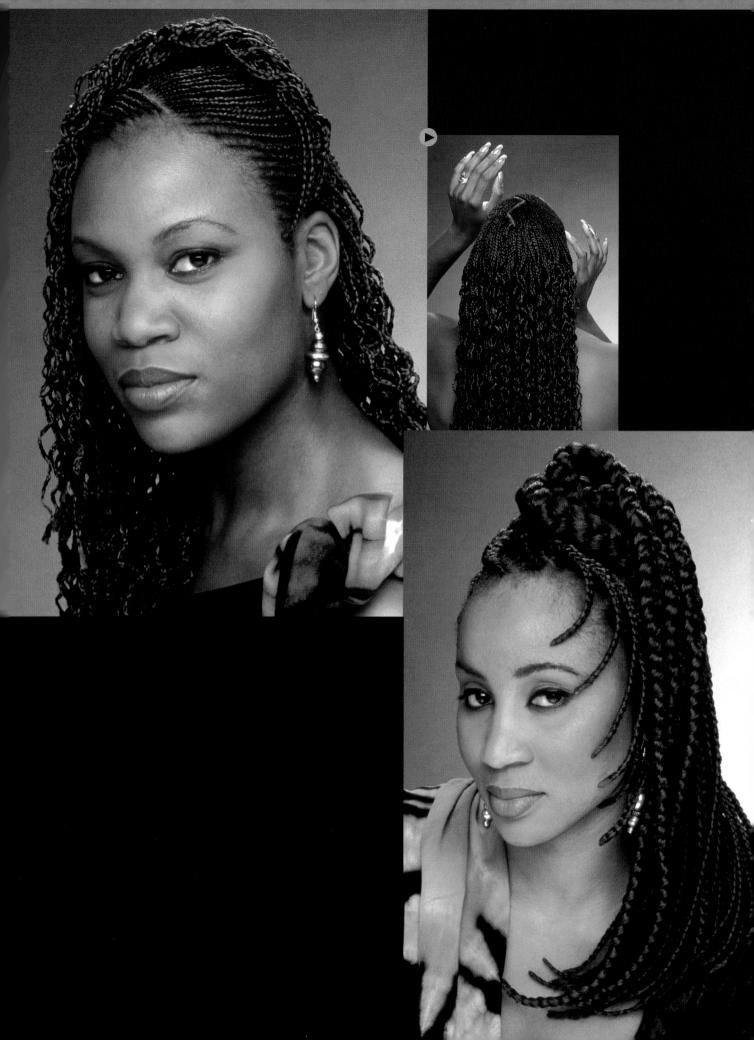

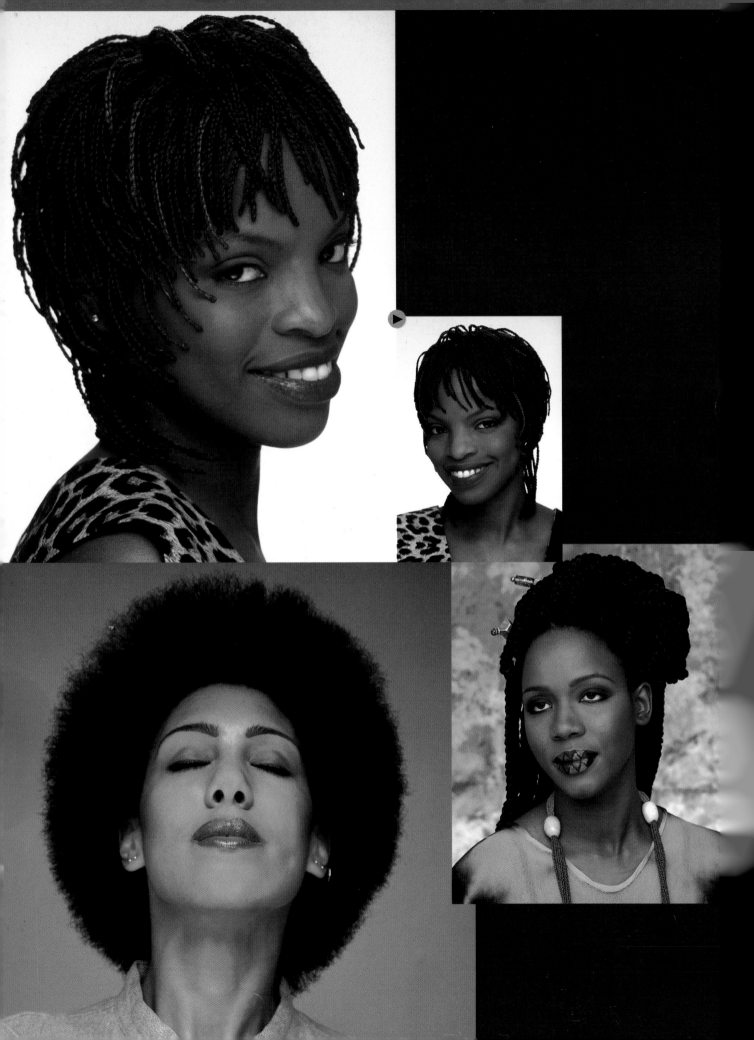